# Medical Radiology

## Diagnostic Imaging

**Series Editors**

Hans-Ulrich Kauczor
Paul M. Parizel
Wilfred C. G. Peh

For further volumes:
http://www.springer.com/series/4354

Carlos Francisco Silva
Oyunbileg von Stackelberg
Hans-Ulrich Kauczor

Editors

# Value-based Radiology

## A Practical Approach

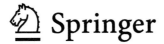 Springer

*Editors*
Carlos Francisco Silva
Diagnostic and Interventional Radiology
University Hospital Heidelberg
Heidelberg, Baden-Württemberg
Germany

Oyunbileg von Stackelberg
Diagnostic and Interventional Radiology
University Hospital Heidelberg
Heidelberg, Baden-Württemberg
Germany

Hans-Ulrich Kauczor
Diagnostic and Interventional Radiology
University Hospital Heidelberg
Heidelberg, Baden-Württemberg
Germany

ISSN 0942-5373          ISSN 2197-4187   (electronic)
Medical Radiology
ISBN 978-3-030-31554-2          ISBN 978-3-030-31555-9   (eBook)
https://doi.org/10.1007/978-3-030-31555-9

This Springer imprint is published by the registered company Springer Nature Switzerland AG
The registered company address is: Gewerbestrasse 11, 6330 Cham, Switzerland

*To my Masters, and to S., my Muse*

– Carlos Francisco Silva

# Preface

Healthcare delivery is experiencing a great transition in terms of "value-based healthcare" or "value-based radiology". The idea behind this transformation is that the providers are paid based on patient's health outcomes and not for the amount of service they delivered. Care for a medical condition usually involves different specialties and a number of interventions, and the value for the patient can only be created by combined efforts of all stakeholders on the entire cycle of care. In this regard, the specialty of radiology is one of the important outcomes influencing players in the whole healthcare cycle, whether contributing to diagnosis, or by minimally invasive interventional procedures, radiation therapy or therapy monitoring. Consequently, radiology departments are facing many challenges to improve operational efficiency, performance and quality to keep pace with this rapid transition in the healthcare delivery. The duty and workload of the radiologist has changed rapidly in the last decades; times when radiologists have analysed "just a film" are long gone. Today, radiologists face an ever increasing workload and yet have to provide the most possible value to the patients, in an adverse context of shortage of imaging specialists and lack of time spent for interpreting and communicating the imaging exams with patients and referring clinicians.

The following issues are inevitable for creating value and contributing to patient outcome in radiology departments.

- well-organized utilization plans for patient scheduling and consequently shorter waiting times for patients;
- guideline compliance, adherence to appropriateness criteria and identification of redundancy;
- accurate and timely exam reporting with adherence to incidental finding reporting criteria, use of standardized lexicon and structured reports;
- proper communication of reports with referring physicians and with patients;
- continuous research for better imaging, intervention and therapy.

The main goal is to achieve a sustainable and affordable care, creating value, better outcomes and satisfaction to both patients and all players in the health cycle.

This book offers a cutting-edge guide to value-based radiology and provides readers with the latest and comprehensive information on all aspects of value-based radiology. All topics are discussed by prominent experts in the field in a clearly organized and illustrated form, which will help readers gain the most from each chapter. Accordingly, the book offers a valuable resource for radiologists and healthcare managers working in public or private institutions, as well as a quick reference guide for all other physicians interested in the topic.

Heidelberg, Baden-Württemberg, Germany                    Carlos Francisco Silva
Heidelberg, Baden-Württemberg, Germany              Oyunbileg von Stackelberg
Heidelberg, Baden-Württemberg, Germany                  Hans-Ulrich Kauczor

# Contents

# Part I

# Theoretical Basis and General Concepts

# Value-Based Radiology: A New Era Begins

Michael Fuchsjäger, Lorenzo Derchi, and Adrian Brady

## Contents

### Abstract

This introduction chapter is written by Prof. Michael Fuchsjäger, Chair of the European Society of Radiology (ESR)'s Value-Based Radiology Subcommittee, Prof. Lorenzo Derchi, Chair of the ESR Board of Directors, and Dr. Adrian Brady, Chair of the ESR Quality, Safety and Standards Committee. Prof. Derchi and Dr. Brady are also ex officio members of the Value-Based Radiology Subcommittee. The Value-Based Radiology Subcommittee was established with the aim of supporting radiologists in fulfilling their central role in healthcare while assisting them in the development of "appropriate metrics, which capture their true contribution and added value to patient care" (European Society of Radiology (ESR), https://www.myesr.org/about/organisation/executive-council#paragraph_grid_16643, Accessed 28 May 2019, 2019). The Subcommittee takes an active role in promoting value-based radiology to patients, through patient groups, and to healthcare professionals, through various publications and other activities, including dedicated sessions and lectures at the European Congress of Radiology (ECR) and stakeholder events such as the ECCO (European CanCer Organisation) summit 2018 and COCIR (European Coordination Committee of the Radiological, Electromedical and Healthcare IT Industry) General Assembly 2018. Furthermore, the Subcommittee collaborates with other radiological societies around the world on various initiatives.

M. Fuchsjäger (✉)
Department of Radiology, Medical University of Graz, Graz, Austria
e-mail: michael.fuchsjaeger@medunigraz.at

L. Derchi
San Martino University of Genoa, Genoa, Italy

A. Brady
Mercy University Hospital, Cork, Ireland

Med Radiol Diagn Imaging (2019)
https://doi.org/10.1007/174_2019_220, © Springer Nature Switzerland AG
Published Online: 08 August 2019

# 1 Introduction

In medical terms, radiology is a young specialty with a relatively short history, beginning with the discovery of X-rays by Wilhelm Conrad Röntgen in 1895. Despite its youth, it has had a transformative impact on the practice of medicine, introducing increasingly complex equipment, capabilities and modalities, and interrupting the direct diagnostic link between physician and patient that had previously existed for millenia (van Gelderen 2004). As a matter of fact, the radiologist's work is now in the middle between the patient and his/her primary care physician, making the patient's body visible and understandable. As radiology has become increasingly technologically sophisticated in recent decades, the distance between patients and radiologists has grown, despite the concomitant growth in the influence of radiology on patient care. Work practices have led to radiologists, with the exception of a few subspecialties (e.g. interventional radiology, breast imaging), retreating to reading rooms, with limited direct patient contact. The rise of teleradiology makes this distance increasingly spatial as well as personal. Consequently, a significant degree exists of ignorance amongst patients about the actual role of the radiologist, as revealed by a 2008 survey conducted by the American College of Radiology (ACR): approximately half of respondents were unable to tell whether radiologists administer or interpret scans nor whether radiologists were licensed physicians or technicians (Glazer and Ruiz-Wibbelsmann 2011).

The increasing digitalisation of radiology has required radiologists to take on an ever-increasing workload: quicker scans and higher patient throughput have resulted in a greater number of examinations and an increased number of images per examination (especially for CT and MRI). Yet the increase in productivity facilitated by improvements in technology has, arguably, only contributed to the increasing commoditisation of radiology as a profession, its work being measured predominantly in terms of volume (Brady 2011a, b). As a matter of fact, it is usually considered that the examinations we perform are fully standardised (as a commodity) and our results are measured predominantly in terms of volume of studies performed. In addition, the current financial difficulties encountered by all healthcare systems and the consequent focus on efficiency make the perception of radiology as nothing more than a numbers game increasingly problematic. Indeed, the question of whether the increasing use of technology such as artificial intelligence (AI) solutions in radiology could make radiologists obsolete has even been raised by some (Ridly 2019; Goedert 2019). The need for radiologists to demonstrate the value that they add to the healthcare value-chain every day has never been more acute.

Value-based healthcare is a conceptualisation of healthcare centred on quality, rather than quantity. It is a response to the increasing costs of healthcare provision, particularly in developed countries. Traditionally, healthcare has focused primarily on responding to acute and emergency episodes. This focus meant there were few incentives for healthcare providers to invest in "prevention, longitudinal chronic disease management, [or] population health" (Philips Position Paper 2019). Furthermore, time-consuming activities such as direct patient consultation were actually dis-incentivised. Value-based healthcare seeks to invert this, placing patients at the centre of the care model.

Value-based healthcare, as a framework, originated in the seminal work of Harvard economist Michael Porter (2010). Its goal is to simultaneously improve health outcomes and reduce costs. By placing patients' outcomes at the centre of the model, value-based healthcare seeks to incentivise improved outcomes for patients instead of merely an increase in workload (including not just potentially unnecessary procedures, but potentially harmful ones) (Kimpen 2019). Specifically, value is defined by Porter as patient health outcome divided by money spent. This formula would suggest two ways of increasing value to patients: either reducing costs for the same outcome, or increasing outcomes relative to costs. This is, of course, not a universally accepted definition of value, the Utah Value in Health Care Survey providing just one example of alternative ways in which value can be assessed (Albo et al. 2018). The European

Commission has convened an expert panel on health, which has produced a draft opinion on value-based healthcare. Their conclusion that value may be measured according to four metrics, personal value ("appropriate care to achieve patients' personal goals" (Expert Panel on Effective Ways of Investigating in Health 2019)), technical value ("achievement of best possible outcomes with available resources" (Expert Panel on Effective Ways of Investigating in Health 2019)), allocative value ("equitable resource distribution across all patient groups" (Expert Panel on Effective Ways of Investigating in Health 2019)), and societal value ("contribution of healthcare to social participation and connectedness" (Expert Panel on Effective Ways of Investigating in Health 2019)), is due to be discussed in June 2019, providing stakeholders, such as radiologists, an opportunity to offer their perspectives.

In the context of the Utah Value in Health Care Survey amongst patients, physicians and employers, University of Utah Health defines value as the "product of the quality of care plus the patient experience at a given cost" (Albo et al. 2018). Thus, University of Utah Health added a subjective element to Porter's value equation by including the service aspect in order to reflect the patient's assessment of value. Adapted to employers, the equation considers employee productivity resulting from better health combined with employee satisfaction, divided by the cost of providing health benefits. One of the main findings of the survey was that patients, physicians, and employers who pay for medical benefits have different opinions of what is most valuable in healthcare. The study's authors therefore conclude that mutual understanding of all stakeholders' positions is a first step towards a value-based healthcare system.

Porter explicitly states that the "proper unit for measuring value should encompass *all services* or activities that jointly determine success in meeting a set of patient needs" (emphasis added) (Porter 2010). Yet, under both the Porter and Utah frameworks, radiology's place in the value chain has, to a large extent, been overlooked thus far. The combined effect of the dislocation of radiologists from patients, a phenomenon Glazer

and Ruiz-Wibbelsmann (2011) describe as leading to the 'invisibility' of radiologists, and the commoditisation of the service they provide has been that diagnosis is not seen as part of the patient health outcome, and radiology is subsequently either absent from the value chain or viewed only as a cost: 'radiology is widely viewed as a contributor to health care costs without an adequate understanding of its contribution to downstream cost savings or improvement in patient outcomes' (Sarwar et al. 2015).

Swift and, above all, accurate diagnosis is irrefutably integral to determining the success of meeting patient needs. Porter himself acknowledges this: "Delays in diagnosis or formulation of treatment plans can cause unnecessary anxiety" (Porter 2010), a factor that would certainly adversely affect value under the subjective element of the University of Utah Health framework. Aside from patient anxiety, it should go without saying that erroneous diagnosis can lead to worse health outcomes, both through failure to optimally treat disease and the performance of unnecessary procedures.

In recent years, radiologists have sought to increase their visibility, for example, through initiatives such as the International Day of Radiology (IDOR) (2019), inaugurated in 2012 by the ESR in association with the Radiological Society of North America (RSNA) and the ACR. IDOR has since become an annual event held with the aim of building greater awareness of the value that radiology contributes to safe patient care, and improving understanding of the vital role radiologists play in the healthcare continuum. IDOR is now celebrated by more than 170 societies all over the world with special publications, social media activities, courses and charity events.

The ESR was amongst the first medical scientific societies to create a patient group (the Patient Advisory Group—PAG) within the society structure, with the specific goal of bringing together "patients, the public and imaging professionals in order to positively influence advances in the field of medical imaging to the benefit of patients in Europe" (European Society of Radiology (ESR) Patient Advisory Group 2019). The ESR-PAG thus serves as a role model for others as it works towards the improvement of radiologist-patient dialogue. The ESR's Value-Based Radiology Subcommittee purposefully included a Patient Advisory Group (PAG) representative with the aim of working with them to boost the visibility of the concept of value-based radiology amongst patients and to consider their perspective.

Other examples of ways radiologists have sought to raise the profile of radiology and build closer connections to patients include informative websites, such as the RSNA and ACR's radiologyinfo.org (Radiology Info 2019), and making increased efforts to routinely speak to patients; Glazer and Ruiz-Wibbelsmann give the examples of personally explaining mammographic results, communicating paediatric imaging results to parents, and utilising online portals to provide enhanced contact with patients (Glazer and Ruiz-Wibbelsmann 2011).

Yet, despite these attempts to make radiology more 'visible', particularly to patients, the precise position of radiology in the value chain remains uncertain as the healthcare industry begins its shift towards value-based metrics (Brandt-Zawadski and Kerlan 2009). As future planning and resource allocation will, more than likely, depend upon such models, it is vital to ensure that radiology's position is recognised. As such, the discussion and perspectives presented in this volume are most welcome, although it should, of course, be noted that the discussion of value-based healthcare and its application to radiology has taken slightly different perspectives on different sides of the Atlantic, largely due to differing models of funding, governance, and payment for healthcare in Europe and the USA (Kimpen 2019), and within different branches of radiology.

## 2    Where Is the Value in Radiology Delivered?

Impact on patients' outcome, and therefore 'value', is delivered in all aspects of radiology, ranging from screening and disease prevention to detection, diagnosis, image-guided biopsy, staging of disease, evaluation of patient progress during treatment, the provision of high-level subspecialist interpretation, reassurance and confirmation of resolution of disease, clinical decision support,

imaging biomarkers, radiation protection, interventional radiology and teleradiology. It is generated by justified indications, appropriate criteria and appropriate dose, personalised patient protocols, structured reporting, reporting of incidental findings, therapeutic decisions based on radiological diagnoses and improved patient outcome. The added value that radiology provides to the healthcare value chain has been documented in various longitudinal studies (Alberle et al. 2013; Mehanna et al. 2016; The SCOT-HEART Investigators 2018). Furthermore, Sarwar et al. (2015) provide a clear illustration of how radiology can deliver value at each step of the imaging chain. Every step of this whole chain can be broken down to several processes, from decision support tools and proper scheduling at the front end, to appropriate communication and follow-up recommendation at the back end. In addition, every process can be measured by specific indicators to help improve practice.

The ESR's 2017 concept paper on value-based radiology (European Society of Radiology (ESR) 2017) adds new aspects to the value chain by identifying five key factors that relate to the quality of the diagnosis and, similar to the University of Utah Health model, focus particularly on the human aspect of the value chain, including the patient's well-being and relations with patients and referring physicians. The first key factor concerns the appropriateness of an imaging request. Clinical decision support systems developed by the radiological community for referring physicians are designed to enhance appropriateness. The ESR's solution is the ESR iGuide (2019), a system for making imaging referral guidelines available to referring physicians at the point of care, providing evidence-based information and decision support. The value of this step consists in ensuring the appropriate use of radiation, avoiding unnecessary exposure and related risks, and contributing to correct protocolling of exams.

Appropriately prioritising patients enables treatment of urgent cases at an early stage, thus reducing patient burden and costs that would be incurred by diagnosis and treatment at a more advanced stage. This enables value to be added during the processes associated with Sarwar et al.'s first step in the value chain (Sarwar et al. 2015).

The second key factor is attention to radiation protection measures. Major radiological societies and organisations have launched radiation protection initiatives, such as ESR EuroSafe Imaging and, following its lead, AFROSAFE, Arab Safe, CanadaSafe, Image Gently, Image Wisely, Japan Safe Imaging, and LATINSAFE. EuroSafe Imaging strives to support and strengthen medical radiation protection across Europe following a holistic, inclusive approach (EuroSafe Imaging 2019), focusing on optimisation, justification, quality and safety, education, research and regulatory compliance. A number of metrics concerning radiation protection should ideally be put in place in every department, for example: the presence of diagnostic protocols which entail the choice of non-ionising examinations whenever possible; the presence of low-dose protocols in all CT equipment; a framework for reporting the percentage of use of such protocols; a requirement to report all exposures to a radiation dose index registry; and training programmes on radiation protection. Visser notes dose monitoring—comparing dosages with diagnostic reference levels (DRLs)—as another step towards ensuring maximum value is provided to patients in terms of safety. Patient preparation, including the choice and administration of contrast media, is another factor that may generate value (Sarwar et al. 2015; Visser 2019).

The third key factor concerns reporting, specifically the characteristics of the radiology report: it should be correct, concise, complete, clearly structured and easily comprehensible to the referring physician (Brady 2018). Following such rules provides value to the referring physician by supplying them with all the information they need to make decisions optimally. Structured reporting will be particularly helpful in the future as it allows the use of decision support tools which can guide the radiologist (Visser 2019). Every radiology report should use standardised terminology, provide specific recommendations about further imaging or treatment, give full contact information, and, ideally, should be made available to the patient via an online portal.

The fourth key factor for adding value is the relationship between patients and radiology personnel. The availability of detailed instructions for different examinations, the distribution of patient satisfaction questionnaires (developed together with PAGs), followed by audits, as well as formal relationships between radiology departments and patient organisations are factors and possible metrics of the radiologist's availability and thus visibility to patients. The importance of this factor to patients was underlined by a survey conducted by the ESR's Value-Based Radiology Subcommittee in 2019 (European Society of Radiology (ESR) 2019b) in which preliminary results indicated that patients in various countries expressed a degree of dissatisfaction with the availability of radiologists for personal consultation, and, to a lesser extent, with both the way their results were communicated to them and the information provided following diagnosis by radiology staff [unpublished]. This is an area in which radiologists may provide significant improvements in perceived value at relatively little expense (assuming sufficient workforce availability).

The fifth key factor according to the ESR concept paper is continuous professional education, research, and innovation. Again, the ESR's Value-Based Radiology Subcommittee's patient survey revealed that a key element that patients regarded as providing value was their confidence in their radiologist's qualifications and expertise. While it is obvious that staying abreast of new developments and using state-of-the-art technology increases value, this factor is particularly difficult to measure. Regarding continuous professional education, compliance with national regulations on continuous medical education (CME) could serve as metrics.

With so many factors through which radiology may contribute to enhancing value for the patient, the referring physician, and health policy makers, it is high time that radiology's place within value-based healthcare models be fully recognised.

## 3 What Is the Status of Value-Based Radiology in Other Parts of the World?

The ESR dedicated its International Forum 2018 to the topic of value-based radiology in an attempt to gain global perspectives on the current status of value-based radiology in different regions and contexts, as well as what efforts are being made to promote value-based radiology. The International Forum is convened annually by the ESR during the ECR and offers the ESR's partner and member societies from outside Europe the opportunity to present the situation regarding a particular topic in their respective country or region. A report on the ESR International Forum 2018 was published in Insights into Imaging in 2019 (European Society of Radiology (ESR) 2019c) and can be summarised as follows:

### North America

In 2017, the Conference Board of Canada, Canada's largest non-partisan, not-for-profit, evidence-based research organisation published a primer document 'The value of radiology in Canada', demonstrating to lawmakers and policymakers that radiology adds value to the health system (The Value of Radiology in Canada 2016). This primer provides three examples: breast cancer screening, teleradiology, and interventional neuroradiology. The Canadian Association of Radiologists (CAR) has been very active in promoting the role of radiology and radiologists through various initiatives designed to raise awareness of who radiologists are, what role they perform, and demonstrate the ways in which radiologists help patients, or improve patients' care in general, e.g. through advocacy activities, such as meetings with stakeholders, or patient care initiatives, such as practice guidelines and various patient resources (European Society of Radiology (ESR) 2019c).

In the United States, the RSNA provides material to enable patients to properly inform themselves about radiology procedures as well as its RadLex and Structured Reporting initiatives to help encourage radiologists to adopt structured and standardised terminology for drafting their reports (Radiological Society of North America 2019). The RSNA takes the perspective that, radiologists can demonstrate the value they add to the patient by taking full responsibility for managing their imaging, thereby assuring the patient that they are fully engaged in their diagnosis/treatment (European Society of Radiology (ESR) 2019c).

The ACR offers its Imaging 3.0 initiative as a roadmap towards value-based imaging, which should be achieved with the help of clinical decision support (CDS), structured reporting, data mining, and other information technology tools (American College of Radiology 2019). Unlike in traditional radiological care, radiologists have to actively take responsibility for all aspects of imaging care, thereby enhancing patients' experience and relevance to the clinical team (European Society of Radiology (ESR) 2019c).

### Latin America

Latin America suffers from considerable disparities in both health and socioeconomic terms between urban and rural areas. Technological developments and value-based radiology initiatives are largely limited to private hospitals. While, overall, efforts still focus on improving access to and coverage of health services rather than on fee for value, the Inter-American College of Radiology (CIR), as well as the major national radiological societies, such as those in Brazil, Colombia, and Mexico, are making efforts to move towards a value-based approach. For example, LATINSAFE is mentioned as an initiative dedicated to education in radiation protection (European Society of Radiology (ESR) 2019c).

**Asia**

In India, like in Latin America, the situation is highly heterogeneous, ranging from modern hospitals with state-of-the-art facilities to villages without any access to imaging whatsoever. According to the Indian Radiological and Imaging Association (IRIA), radiologists should be perceived as clinicians interacting with their patients. In Korea, the government has increased the budget for assessing and increasing medical quality, and the Korean Society of Radiology (KSR) embraces the value-based healthcare system. The Japan Radiological Society (JRS) launched Japan Safe Radiology, a government-supported project to promote safety, standardisation and optimisation of imaging, and plans to add value-based radiology to the project's safety and efficiency related targets (European Society of Radiology (ESR) 2019c).

Asia-Oceania is yet another region where the practice of value-based radiology is very diverse. In most countries, radiology departments are seen primarily as service providers, with turnaround times of reports still viewed as the key indicator. However, some moves are being made towards value-based metrics: Choosing Wisely Australia is a clinician-led global initiative aiming to improve safety and quality in healthcare by avoiding unnecessary examinations, treatments and procedures (Choosing Wisely Australia 2019). With InsideRadiology, the Royal Australian and New Zealand College of Radiologists (RANZCR) offers patients and referring physicians information on clinical radiology tests, treatments and procedures (Inside Radiology 2019). Furthermore, RANZCR offers educational modules to promote appropriateness of referrals (European Society of Radiology (ESR) 2019c).

To summarise, although the extent to which value-based radiology has been adopted still varies between countries and within countries, the world's major radiological societies agree that the value-based approach is the concept to follow in the future.

## 4 Perspective

Radiology has finally begun to appreciate that the quality and the value it provides is more important than the mere volume, previously the main driver of and unit used for measuring productivity and efficacy. As in healthcare as a whole, radiology will in future be measured according to patient outcome, which will certainly be better with the improving quality and safety of the entire imaging chain: decision to image, performance of procedure, interpretation of study, reporting of study, and the highly important last step of communication of results to our patients and referring physicians.

Change is inevitable in healthcare, especially in specialities which rely heavily on technology, such as radiology. Radiologists must continue to show themselves to be adaptable and willing to change: it is the only way to survive evolutionary processes, and emerge stronger and better. The evolution which this new era of value-based radiology ushers in is an opportunity to enhance the ability of radiologists to provide the best possible care for patients and secure their position at the heart of ensuring optimum outcomes.

To accomplish all this in the near future the role and—very importantly—the self-image of the radiologist will have to change considerably: from that of the traditional image interpreter to that of the leader of the whole imaging process, and perhaps even of integrated diagnostics in the more distant future. Accepting this new role entails accepting heightened responsibility as a large number of processes—many of which have been managed separately by radiology for a long time—have to be integrated into one cohesive body around the framework of value-based radiology.

The more active role of radiologists in creating value will necessarily include a better understanding for the needs of the referral base through active engagement with referring physicians, for example, having daily consultations with subspecialties within the department or embedding reading rooms in specialty clinics of referring physicians and, obviously, improving radiology reports themselves with regard to structure and standardisation.

Artificial Intelligence (AI) will undoubtedly play a role in this. Currently, AI seems to show most promise in certain specific fields or niches, e.g. helping with repetitive tasks like lesion detection and feature description; it has also offered potential as a decision support tool (Savadjiev et al. 2019). This could be of vital importance in the future as AI frees time for interpretation and communication and/or makes coping with the ever-increasing workload possible, especially in regions where radiologists are scarce (teleradiology could also play a vital role here). In short, AI offers radiologists further potential to generate increased value. Rather than seeing AI as an existential threat (Ridly 2019; Goedert 2019), radiologists should embrace AI as an additional means through which they can enhance value to patients (e.g. by using deep learning to lower dosage for CT scans) (Visser 2019).

## 5   Conclusion

At the end of the day, each radiologist has to provide the best possible care for his/her patients; therefore, any definition of the "value" provided by our work should rightly be focused on patient outcome. For all patients, radiology can have impact in different moments of each episode of care, thus continuously providing value and contributing to patient outcome. Furthermore, such contributions are extremely broad and involve well-managed imaging utilisation plans, shortening of waiting times for imaging exams, improved appropriateness, attention to radiation protection, use of structured reporting, using the 'drivers seat' position in introducing technological

innovation including AI tools and solutions to improve diagnostic imaging, interventional radiology and image-guide therapy. However, the two most crucial aspects through which we add value to patient outcome remain close collaboration with our referring physicians and communication with our patients. As regards the first, liaising with colleagues and working together as a team, both informally and in regular multidisciplinary meetings, is the basis of appropriate use of imaging as well as of correct therapeutic choices based on the resulting images. As regards the latter, communication with patients not only makes radiologists 'visible', but contributes to giving radiology the prominence its importance to value-based healthcare deserves.

**Acknowledgements** The authors acknowledge and thank the following individuals for their particular contributions: Jonathan Clark, Martina Szucsich, and Monika Hierath (ESR Department of European & International Affairs).

## References

Alberle DR, DeMello S, Berg CD et al (2013) Results of the two incidence screenings in national lung screening trial. N Engl J Med 369(10):920–931

Albo A, Bracken S, Orlandi R et al (2018) Bringing value into focus: the state of value in U.S. Health Care. University of Utah Health, Salt Lake City, UT

American College of Radiology (2019) Imaging 3.0. https://www.acr.org/Practice-Management-Quality-Informatics/Imaging-3. Accessed 6 Jun 2019

Brady AP (2011a) Measuring radiologist workload: how to do it, and why it matters. Eur Radiol 21(11):2315–2317

Brady AP (2011b) Measuring consultant radiologist workload: method and results from a national survey. Insights Imaging 2:247–260

Brady AP (2018) Radiology reporting—from Hemingway to HAL? Insights Imaging 9:237–246

Brandt-Zawadski M, Kerlan RK (2009) Patient-centered radiology: use it or lose it! Acad Radiol 16:521–523

Choosing Wisely Australia (2019). http://www.choosingwisely.org.au/home. Accessed 6 Jun 2019

ESR iGuide (2019). https://www.myesr.org/esriguide. Accessed 3 Jun 2019

European Society of Radiology (ESR) (2017) ESR concept paper on value-based radiology. Insights Imaging 8:447–454

European Society of Radiology (ESR) (2019a). https://www.myesr.org/about/organisation/executive-council#paragraph_grid_16643. Accessed 28 May 2019

European Society of Radiology (ESR) (2019b) Value-based radiology subcommittee patient survey. https://www.myesr.org/esr-patient-survey-value-based-radiology. Accessed 20 May 2019

European Society of Radiology (ESR) (2019c) Summary of the proceedings of the international forum 2018: "value-based radiology". Insights Imaging 10:34

European Society of Radiology (ESR) Patient Advisory Group (2019). https://www.myesr.org/sites/default/files/ESR-PAG-leaflet-web.pdf. Accessed 3 Jun 2019

EuroSafe Imaging (2019). http://www.eurosafeimaging.org/about. Accessed 21 May 2019

Expert Panel on Effective Ways of Investigating in Health (2019) Opinion on defining value in 'value-based healthcare'. https://ec.europa.eu/health/expert_panel/sites/expertpanel/files/024_valuebasedhealthcare_en.pdf. Accessed 3 Jun 2019

Glazer GM, Ruiz-Wibbelsmann JA (2011) The invisible radiologist. Radiology 258:18–22

Goedert J (2019) Are radiologists becoming obsolete? https://www.healthdatamanagement.com/news/are-radiologists-becoming-obsolete. Accessed 23 May 2019

Inside Radiology (2019). https://www.insideradiology.com.au/. Accessed 6 Jun 2019

International Day of Radiology (2019). https://www.internationaldayofradiology.com/. Accessed 24 May 2019

Kimpen J (2019) How health care informatics supports increased productivity and better patient experiences. https://www.politico.eu/sponsored-content/how-health-care-informatics-supports-increased-productivity-and-better-patient-experiences/. Accessed 21 May 2019

Mehanna H, Wong W-L, McConkey CC et al (2016) PET-CT surveillance versus neck dissection in advanced head and neck cancer. N Engl J Med 374:1444–1454

Philips Position Paper (2019) Value-based care: turning healthcare theory into a dynamic and patient-focused reality. https://www.philips.com/a-w/about/news/archive/blogs/innovation-matters/20190212-how-informatics-supports-increased-productivity-better-outcomes-and-improved-experiences-in-healthcare.html. Accessed 20 May 2019

Porter EM (2010) What is value in healthcare? N Engl J Med 363:26

Radiological Society of North America (2019) RadLex radiology lexicon. https://www.rsna.org/en/practice-tools/data-tools-and-standards/radlex-radiology-lexicon. Accessed 6 Jun 2019

Radiology Info (2019). https://www.radiologyinfo.org/. Accessed 3 Jun 2019

Ridly EL (2019) Will AI soon put radiologists out of a job? https://www.auntminnie.com/index.aspx?sec=sup&sub=aic&pag=dis&ItemID=114604. Accessed 22 May 2019

Sarwar A, Boland G, Monks A et al (2015) Metrics for radiologists in the era of value-based health care delivery. Radiographics 35:866–878

Savadjiev P, Chong J, Dohan A et al (2019) Demystification of AI-driven medical image interpretation: past, present and future. Eur Radiol 29:1616–1624

The SCOT-HEART Investigators (2018) Coronary CT angiography and 5-year risk of myocardial infarction. N Engl J Med 379:924–933

The Value of Radiology in Canada (2016) The Conference Board of Canada. https://www.conferenceboard.ca/temp/9a7de99e-3869-4676-addd-823dedcb3968/8532_ValueofRadiology_BR_.pdf. Accessed 6 Jun 2019

van Gelderen F (2004) Understanding X-rays. Springer, Berlin

Visser JJ (2019) EuSoMII Webinar Series 2019 'Value based Imaging'. https://www.eusomii.org/6496-2/. Accessed 22 May 2019

# Patient-Centered Care

Carlos Francisco Silva, Kheng L. Lim,
Teresa Guerra, Gianluca Ficarra,
and Ricarda von Krüchten

## Contents

C. F. Silva (✉) · R. von Krüchten
Department of Diagnostic and Interventional
Radiology, University Hospital Heidelberg,
Heidelberg, Germany
e-mail: Carlos.dasilva@med.uni-heidelberg.de

K. L. Lim
Department of Radiology, Pennsylvania Hospital,
University of Pennsylvania Health System,
Philadelphia, PA, USA

T. Guerra
IMA—Imagens Médicas Associadas, Setúbal, Portugal

G. Ficarra
Department of Diagnostic and Interventional
Radiology, University Hospital Heidelberg,
Heidelberg, Germany

Department of Diagnostic and Interventional Radiology,
University of Genoa Hospital, Genoa, Italy

## Abstract

In this chapter we focus on the topics of patient-centered care, or more broadly speaking patient- and family-centered care. The various aspects of improving patient experience in healthcare are discussed. These include patient comfort in a healthcare facility, surveying patients of the care they receive, patient education and providing compassion in delivering bad news, and involvement of patient social circles, among others. A five-step approach in communicating bad news is discussed. In addition, we highlight the importance of promoting the well-being of healthcare providers and its impact on improving patient health outcomes.

## 1 Introduction

Patient-centered care, or more inclusively patient- and family-centered care (PFCC), is generating lots of discussion and gaining momentum in the medical community, especially in the last 5 years. In this model, healthcare delivery revolves around the patient with the emphasis on generating a more pleasant experience from the patient perspective (Itri 2015). In radiology, this includes but is not

Med Radiol Diagn Imaging (2019)
https://doi.org/10.1007/174_2019_209, © Springer Nature Switzerland AG
Published Online: 24 May 2019

limited to timely scheduling of exams, efficient registration, compassionate and knowledgeable staff, peaceful and comfortable environment, radiologist expertise, timely reports, radiologist availability for consultation with the patients and referring physicians, and transparent billing with easy accessibility when questions arise. As patient experience gains traction in influencing reimbursement for health services, it is more important than ever that physicians adopt PFCC paradigm. Radiology consult is discussed separately on the next chapter. Here we discuss the access and waiting times (patient comfort), the involvement of family and friends, the patient education (fear and anxiety alleviation), and finally the PFCC model coexistence with the triple/quadruple aim.

## 2 Access and Waiting Times: Patient Comfort

In a recent study published by Boos et al., it was found that cleanliness, waiting time, patient-staff communication, and especially courtesy of the receptionist were the most important factors for patient satisfaction (Boos et al. 2017). In their tertiary-care academic radiology department, they analyzed patient satisfaction surveys obtained either via online or via electronic kiosks. Interestingly, electronic kiosks generated higher patient response rates than online surveys (92.4% vs. 7.6%; $p < 0.001$), and the location of the electronic kiosks (Fig. 1) also influenced the patient response rates which were found to be lower in changing and waiting areas compared to those next to elevators (63.8% vs. 77.8%; $p < 0.0001$) (Boos et al. 2017).

The importance of a good design in the radiology department environment was demonstrated by Holbrook et al. in their study showing that patients underestimated waiting times when the environment was specifically designed to optimize the patient experience (Holbrook et al. 2016). Their outpatient waiting room was set very well with the ultimate patient experience in mind: ample reading materials, multiple large-

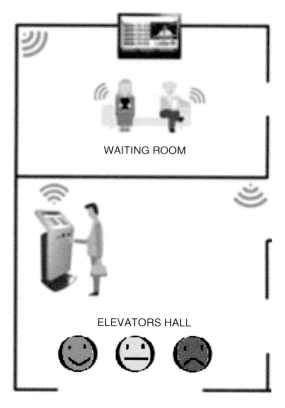

**Fig. 1** Electronic kiosks have become very popular nowadays with their colored faces on the screens, and are becoming popular also in imaging facilities. The best location is probably near the elevators or the exit [adapted by permission from Springer Nature: Serapicos M., Peixoto H., Alves V. (2017) A Hospital Service Kiosk in the Patient's Pocket. In: De Paz J., Julián V., Villarrubia G., Marreiros G., Novais P. (eds) Ambient Intelligence–Software and Applications – eighth International Symposium on Ambient Intelligence (ISAmI 2017). ISAmI 2017. Advances in Intelligent Systems and Computing, vol 615. Springer, Cham. DOI: 10.1007/978-3-319-61118-1_27]

screen televisions (Fig. 2), free Wi-Fi, periodic offer of progress updates, warm blankets, and drinks by the team members, as well as electronic tablet devices (with games and Internet access), were the main components of this exquisite environment. In the end, shorter wait times were, as expected, associated with higher satisfaction scores, and the difference between perceived total waiting time and the actual interval between arrival time and exam start was statistically significant ($p < 0.001$) (Holbrook et al. 2016).

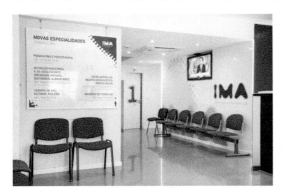

**Fig. 2** Large-screen televisions and free Wi-Fi are good options to optimize the patient experience. Perceived shorter waiting times are associated with higher satisfaction scores

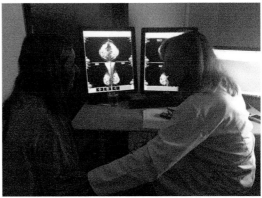

**Fig. 3** Many different activities to promote emotional support for the patient can be performed, such as touching the patient on the hand or arm while giving bad news (Farber et al. 2002). Depicted in this figure: a face-to-face interaction between a patient and Dr. Teresa Guerra (with permission)

## 3    Patient Education: Fear and Anxiety Alleviation

Patients are increasingly accessing Internet-based resources to obtain information about radiologic procedures they are to undergo. In order to make information about diagnostic and interventional procedures in radiology easily accessible from a single source, the Radiological Society of North America (RSNA) and the American College of Radiology (ACR) developed a website (RadiologyInfo 2018) for the public, explaining in lay terms the various diagnostic and interventional procedures using various imaging modalities such as X-ray, CT, MRI, ultrasound, and nuclear medicine, as well as a section for radiation therapy. *RadiologyInfo.org* website currently contains information of over 240 procedures, exams, and disease descriptions which can be viewed in English or Spanish.

Besides interventional and pediatric radiology perhaps there is no subspecialty in radiology more prone to patient and family anxiety like breast imaging, as breast cancer is a very sensitive, high-rated, and mediatic issue. Just take the example of the monetary reimbursement for a low-dose CT scan for lung cancer screening in the United States: less than half for a mammogram (ACR 2018).

As physicians, diagnostic radiologists can create opportunities for patient interactions and therefore can be instrumental in guiding the patient through the medical maze. Interventional radiologists are long known to have face-to-face interactions with patients due to the nature of their work, but radiologists specialized in breast imaging are in unique position to offer compassionate care and provide emotional support to patients when conveying bad news.

One study showed that in breast cancer survivors, anticipatory anxiety and pain catastrophizing were associated with a higher rate of not returning for mammograms (Shelby et al. 2012). Another study (Harvey et al. 2007) laid out a five-step approach in communicating bad news for radiologists specializing in breast imaging:

– Preparing for the encounter
– Disclosing the news
– Evaluating the patient's response
– Discussing the next step
– Offering support (Fig. 3)

Even in the setting when a biopsy of a breast lesion yields benign results, there can still be high psychological burden in women. This does diminish with time but does not completely resolve (Schonberg et al. 2014). We recommend that the breast radiologist should convey the good news first to immediately relieve the anxiety, so that women will be better able to focus on further instructions.

## 4    Involvement of Family and Friends

Social support is a well-known, if not the most important, factor affecting one's life satisfaction. Social support is particularly important when one faces adversities such as significant health morbidities which result in disability or significant change in lifestyle. Therefore, it is no surprise that patients will often share the diagnosis of their health calamities with family members and close friends. As the delivery of healthcare evolves, the inclusion of people important to the patients proves to be beneficial in affecting the outcomes of care. Besides tissue diagnosis of diseases, radiologists are often in a position to make the initial diagnosis through imaging, and at times a near-certain diagnosis of diseases including malignancy. Therefore, radiologists can improve the quality of care and patient satisfaction by including family members when providing information about imaging procedures or discussing abnormal findings (Itri 2015).

Harrison and Frampton (2016) argue that research design should also include engagement with patients and their families in an era of paradigm shift where patients are asked the question of "what matters most."

> **Key Points**
> - **New PFCC (patient- and family-centered care) practices to pursue in radiology:** Patient comfort, e.g., access and waiting times in imaging facilities, patient education, fear and anxiety alleviation, and involvement of all the stakeholders such as friends and caregivers.
> - **Increase visibility, increase value:** Expanding the traditional field and tasks of radiology, like actively pursuing these PFCC practices, may be the most valuable weapon to fight the threat of commoditization of medical imaging.

## 5    The Quadruple Aim and the PFCC Model Coexistence

In the United States, a nonprofit, private organization called the National Committee for Quality Assurance (NCQA) provides accreditation and the "gold seal" for high-quality practices. NCQA started its model of high-quality care organizing around primary care in 2008, and in 2013 it broadened its scope to involve specialty practices called Patient-Centered Specialty Practice (PCSP) (NCQA 2018; Greene et al. 2017). The NCQA PCSP model has six pillars (NCQA 2018) that describe the core components of the PFCC framework:

- Provide access/communication
- Identify patient populations
- Track and coordinate referrals
- Plan and manage care
- Track and coordinate care
- Measure and improve performance

Greene et al. illustrated the practical application of this model in the daily clinical practice of radiologists. Although the NCQA PCSP guidelines are well intended, the cost associated with implementation of new activities and the lack of increased payment from payers to offset the cost pose a real-life challenge (Greene et al. 2017). More rules and regulations can have unintended side effects to the medical practitioners. Increased bureaucracy without corresponding increase in clerical and other ancillary support can fuel job dissatisfaction and potentially lead to burnout.

Much debate has emerged in the last decade about the *Triple Aim in Healthcare* and using PFCC practices to achieve it. The Triple Aim was envisioned by Donald Berwick a decade ago (Berwick et al. 2008) to improve the patient experience of care, improve the health of populations, and reduce the cost of healthcare. Since then, with increasing reliance on metrics and methods to reduce cost, health practitioners are constantly under the pressure to increase productivity. The pursuit to maintain profitability by administrators and managers in the healthcare business also trickles down to the practitioners to treat more patients and perform more procedures. Bodenheimer et al. reminded us that there must be a fourth aim to balance the goals of the Triple Aim, i.e., to consider the well-being of health practitioners at and off work while keeping patient interest at the center of care (Bodenheimer and Sinsky 2014). This fourth aim was recently recognized and incorporated into the Declaration of Geneva (Hippocratic Oath) by the World Medical Association in 2017. The new sentence is "I will attend to my own health, well-being, and abilities in order to provide care of the highest standard" (BioEdge 2018; Parsa-Parsi 2017).

As the topic of physician burnout gains more attention in the lay media, a recent meta-analysis by Panagioti et al. in 2018 showed that the issue of physician burnout has trickle-down effect and may jeopardize patient care (Panagioti et al. 2018). In their analysis, patient safety incidents and suboptimal care owing to low professionalism were twice as likely to be related with burnout physicians, while receiving low satisfaction ratings from patients was three times more likely to occur with those affected physicians (Panagioti et al. 2018). Because of this untoward effect, Panagioti et al. suggested that healthcare organizations should invest in efforts to improve physician wellness, particularly for early-career physicians.

Radiologists are no exception to burnout. In fact, burnout in radiology was ranked above average when compared to other specialties. As physician burnout becomes more transparent in the medical community, some authors propose a seven-step solution which they call the *Road to Wellness* (Fishman et al. 2018). This includes acknowledging the problem, leadership commitment, finding solutions inside and outside of the workplace, and mindfulness of all involved. Engagement in leisure and outdoor activities, group relaxation practices, and social events with colleagues are some techniques to mitigate burnout (Fishman et al. 2018).

> **Key Points**
> - **The (original) Triple Aim in Healthcare:** improving the outcomes: (1) patient health, (2) patient satisfaction; and (3) reducing the costs.
> - **The (modern) Quadruple Aim in Healthcare:** the mental and physical well-being of the physicians and other healthcare practitioners should be considered while improving the patient experience of care, improving the health of populations, and reducing the cost of healthcare.
> - **Hippocratic Oath (2017 version), NEW:** "I will attend to my own health, well-being, and abilities in order to provide care of the highest standard."

## 6 Summary

Medicine is in an era of transitioning from old practice of "paternalistic" medicine to modern practice where patients participate fully in their healthcare. PFCC practices are becomingly more mainstream and it is imperative for radiology practice to adapt as patients now have more choices than ever. This paradigm shift includes all facets of physician-patient encounter that can bring added value such as from the ease of scheduling an appointment, office visit and facility amenities, diagnostic testing, patient education, and active inclusion of all stakeholders important to the patient (family, friends, caregivers, etc.). The radiology profession should position itself to embark on this journey and actively participate in improving patient experience beyond generating imaging reports. In striving to achieve optimal experience, it should be noted that not all requests from patients are reasonable and some expectations can potentially be detrimental to health providers and their staff. Therefore, PFCC practices should be inclusive of everyone, and we should be mindful in balancing the experience of patients and healthcare providers. Best health practices cannot be achieved by adopting a one-way street; best practices stem from mutual respect, mindfulness, and innate desire to help those in needs.

## References

ACR (2018). https://www.acr.org/Media-Center/ACR-News-Releases/2018/Nelson-Lung-Cancer-Screening-Study-Confirms-NLST-Results (Accessed 18 December 2018)

Berwick DM, Nolan TW, Whittington J (2008) The Triple Aim: care, health, and cost. Health Aff (Millwood) 27(3):759–769

BioEdge (2018). https://www.bioedge.org/bioethics/new-hippocratic-oath-for-doctors-approved/12496. Accessed 9 December 2018

Bodenheimer T, Sinsky C (2014) From triple to quadruple aim: care of the patient requires care of the provider. Ann Fam Med 12(6):573–576

Boos J, Fang J, Snell A et al (2017) Electronic kiosks for patient satisfaction survey in radiology. AJR Am J Roentgenol 208(3):577–584

Farber NJ, Urban SY, Collier VU et al (2002) The good news about giving bad news to patients. J Gen Intern Med 17(12):914–922

Fishman MDC, Mehta TS, Siewert B et al (2018) The road to wellness: engagement strategies to help radiologists achieve joy at work. Radiographics 38(6):1651–1664

Greene AM, Bailey CR, Young M et al (2017) Applying the National Committee for quality assurance patient-centered specialty practice framework to radiology. J Am Coll Radiol 14(9):1173–1176

Harrison J, Frampton S (2016 Dec) Patient and family engagement in research in era 3. J Am Coll Radiol 13(12 Pt B):1622–1624

Harvey JA, Cohen MA, Brenin DR et al (2007) Breaking bad news: a primer for radiologists in breast imaging. J Am Coll Radiol 4(11):800–808

Holbrook A, Glenn H Jr, Mahmood R et al (2016) Shorter perceived outpatient MRI wait times associated with higher patient satisfaction. J Am Coll Radiol 13(5):505–509

Itri JN (2015) Patient-centered radiology. Radiographics 35(6):1835–1846

NCQA (2018). http://go.nationalpartnership.org/site/DocServer/NCQA.SPR.FactSheet.2012.pdf?docID=11461. Accessed 9 December 2018

Panagioti M, Geraghty K, Johnson J et al (2018) Association between physician burnout and patient safety, professionalism, and patient satisfaction: a systematic review and meta-analysis. JAMA Intern Med 178:1317–1330

Parsa-Parsi RW (2017) The revised declaration of Geneva: a modern-day physician's pledge. JAMA 318(20):1971–1972

RadiologyInfo (2018) (http://www.radiologyinfo.org). Accessed 9 December 2018

Schonberg MA, Silliman RA, Ngo LH et al (2014) Older women's experience with a benign breast biopsy—a mixed methods study. J Gen Intern Med 29(12):1631–1640

Shelby RA, Scipio CD, Somers TJ et al (2012) Prospective study of factors predicting adherence to surveillance mammography in women treated for breast cancer. J Clin Oncol 30(8):813–819

# The Radiology Consult

Carlos Francisco Silva, Claus Peter Heussel,
and Eduardo Mortani Barbosa Jr.

## Contents

C. F. Silva
Department of Diagnostic and Interventional
Radiology, Translational Lung Research Center
(TLRC), German Lung Research Center (DZL),
University Hospital of Heidelberg,
Heidelberg, Germany

C. P. Heussel
Department of Diagnostic and Interventional
Radiology with Nuclear Medicine, Translational
Lung Research Center (TLRC), German Lung
Research Center (DZL), Thoraxklinik GmbH at
University Hospital of Heidelberg,
Heidelberg, Germany

E. Mortani Barbosa Jr. (✉)
Director of Thoracic CT, Department of Radiology,
University of Pennsylvania, Philadelphia, PA, USA
e-mail: Eduardo.Barbosa@uphs.upenn.edu

## Abstract

A rise in radiology consult, in parallel with an ever-growing offer of value-based services, is currently increasing patient awareness of the radiologist's role in clinical care. A German and a North American example of radiology consult are shown in this chapter. The German example, taken from the Radiology Department of the Thoraxklinik University Heidelberg, chaired by Prof. Dr. Claus Peter Heussel, will show different aspects like the workflow regarding severely immunocompromised patients being submitted to thoracic CT, the image-guided biopsy and re-biopsy of nodules or masses, regular tumor boards, and the Interstitial Lung Disease multidisciplinary conference (with pneumologist, radiologist, and pathologist). The University of Pennsylvania at Philadelphia embedded thoracic radiology reading room within an integrated Lung Center Clinic, is the North American example. A survey taken in this large tertiary academic medical center by Dr. Mortani Barbosa Jr. found an overwhelming positive response from the referring healthcare providers, and major positive impact on patient care and management. The most common reasons for consultation were to clarify interpretation of imaging studies and diagnoses, to assess for temporal changes, and in up to 25% of the cases to discuss management options. The radiology consult models we proposed can be implemented in most

Med Radiol Diagn Imaging (2019)
https://doi.org/10.1007/174_2019_208, © Springer Nature Switzerland AG
Published Online: 02 July 2019

mid- to large-size hospitals. The radiologist as a consultant should be seen as the future but also a return to a past in which the interaction of radiologists and referring practitioners was the foundation of diagnosis and medical decision-making.

# 1 Introduction

Last years have witnessed the rise of radiology consult in parallel with the growing offer of value-based services, increasing patient awareness of the radiologist's role in clinical care (Mangano et al. 2015; Gunn et al. 2015; Mortani Barbosa and Novak 2018). Wider availability and lower patient burden (short scan time resulting in seconds of breath-hold, lower radiation dose, and lower costs) caused higher acceptance of radiological services by patients. Joint image result interpretation together with the clinician taking the recent treatment into account to measure, i.e., oncological response, differential diagnosis including organ toxicities, and pseudo-progression, led to a higher value of imaging. Communication of examination findings directly to patients, explanation of interventional radiological procedures, and follow-up of these interventions are among the most frequent in breast, thoracic, and interventional radiology. These value added actions will probably survive the wide introduction of artificial intelligence applications in the radiological specialty. A European and a North American perspective of the pivotal aspects of the radiology consult are reviewed.

# 2 Radiology Consult: The Thoraxklinik Heidelberg Experience

The practice of patient-centered care at the Radiology Department of Thoraxklinik University Heidelberg, chaired by Prof. Dr. Claus Peter Heussel, could be dated back to the 1990s when Heussel locally pioneered a workflow regarding severely immunocompromised patients being submitted to thoracic CT (Heussel et al. 1997) instead of chest X-ray alone as done in immunocompetent ones. These immunocompromised patients deserved special attention, and as such a multidisciplinary discussion was set with the hemato-oncology team, regarding every single patient unique clinical features. Clearly a "one-size-fits-all" policy was not appropriate for the whole radiological care that was given to these frail patients, encompassing varied aspects such as CT protocol, reading, reporting, and communication. This workflow was well taken by clinicians and became standard of care nowadays.

Since the beginning of this century, the image-guided biopsy of nodules or masses was becoming more and more frequent. Nowadays, re-biopsy of known tumors is adding further requests to interventional radiologists, as microbiological changes during treatment require additional attention. Therefore, a dedicated workflow was also set in motion since then. Every single patient that is submitted to interventional procedures in this department is beforehand subject to an interview with the attending thoracic radiologist that is going to ultimately perform the intervention on that respective patient. This establishes a personal relation between the interventional radiologist and patient, who later has to cooperate during the intervention as anesthesia is done locally only. Patients are presented with their own personal radiological findings on workstation screens (Fig. 1), which increases the awareness, motivation, and confidence for the intervention that will be performed.

A thorough explanation about the risks is given to every patient, including the major—pneumothorax, bleeding, death, stroke, and infection—as well as pertaining to patient anticoagulation, and of course about the benefits and safety of such procedures. In our experience, not a single patient that at the beginning was reluctant to being submitted to a biopsy or ablation remained reluctant or refused to do so after this consultation. After this informed consent, an informed consent is signed by both, and the patient is handed a copy including a self-explanatory CT image of the procedure, as well as a plan for which drug to continue or to stop (anticoagulation), when to stop eating, when to appear in the hospital for the intervention, etc.

Besides regular tumor boards, which are nowadays integrated in all comprehensive cancer centers, the Interstitial Lung Disease (ILD) multidisciplinary conference (pneumologist, radiologist, pathologist) has been implemented. It takes place every week (Fig. 2), and that dates back to 2011 approximately, and we must say that once again the patient is the center of the care (Jo et al. 2016). We also have interdisciplinary conferences at the University of Pennsylvania for ILD and oncologic patients.

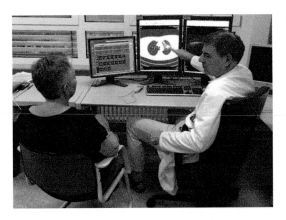

**Fig. 1** A photo showing a radiology consult at Thoraxklinik Heidelberg. Prof. Dr. Claus Peter Heussel explains the patient where the nodule is located in her lung (with permission)

Every single case or thoracic CT is discussed with the referring pneumologist on site, and the patient (although not present in the room) knows precisely that his/her condition or disease is being submitted to a multispecialty analysis (pneumologist, radiologist, pathologist, thoracic surgeon, oncologist, radiation therapist) on that day, with the radiologist being a pivotal asset to assist the referring physician in the diagnosis and management of his/her illness. The protocol thereof becomes part of the patient's record and is therefore transparent for patient and the entire treatment personnel.

## 3 The University of Pennsylvania Embedded Thoracic Radiology Reading Room Within an Integrated Lung Center Clinic

### 3.1 Background

In the United States, current decentralized healthcare reimbursement models compensate medical services through a resource-based relative value scale that assigns an arbitrary number of relative value units (RVUs) to every medical procedure or service, coded utilizing a system called current procedural terminology (CPT), in conjunction

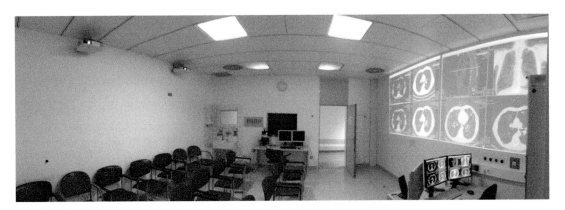

**Fig. 2** A panoramic view of the multidisciplinary conference room at the Thoraxklinik. Two projectors held on the ceiling give the medical audience an excellent detail of what is depicted on the two radiologist's high-resolution monitors. In the center of the image is also shown the microscope and two small monitors for the pathologist. As the microscope can also be connected to one of the projectors, we can show microscopic and radiologic image side by side. Also clinical images (endoscopy, reports, lung function, etc.) can be shown side by side

with ICD-10 diagnostic codes. Each RVU has a monetary value that includes physician effort, practice costs, and geographic differences. This system is the so-called *fee-for-service* model, which strongly incentivizes volume and explicitly neither takes into consideration the quality of the services, nor patient outcomes.

Until recently, there were virtually no mechanisms to reward quality. In other words, the focus has historically been in producing more services, especially expensive ones, with little if any concern regarding the impact on patient outcomes or population health, therefore with little concern for value. We believe that the current US payment system is on an unsustainable course, given progressively rising costs to care for an aging population, and as physicians we ought to provide the highest possible value to society at large but at a reasonable cost, which necessarily implies making quality a centerpiece of future reimbursement models, at the same time we rein in costs. Measuring and promoting quality is not straightforward; however radiology can and should have a leading role in that endeavor.

Radiologists have traditionally practiced in relative isolation from other physicians, relying on their final product—the radiology report—as a means of communication with patients and referring physicians. While this is necessary for reimbursement and documentation, it is not sufficient to maximize our impact and the value we provide. Modern practice of medicine necessitates collaborative multidisciplinary discussions, and radiologists must become active consultants, providing useful guidance and assistance, to ensure our continued relevance in medicine. As we transition to value-based care, radiologists must seek out ways to provide value beyond just generating a written report, by contributing to better quality patient care and outcomes, at a lower total cost. This can be done via in-person consultations, potentially conveying better information in a bidirectional fashion. How can this be accomplished in a busy, complex clinical environment? At the University of Pennsylvania, a large tertiary academic medical center in the Northeastern United States, we established a multidisciplinary Lung Center Clinic (LCC) encompassing clinic space and time for physicians seeing patients with thoracic diseases, with an integrated,

centrally located, radiology reading room staffed by thoracic radiologists and trainees throughout regular working hours (8 am to 5 pm), in which referring physicians can easily walk in at any time, without any appointment or bureaucracy, for in-person consultations. Sometimes, the patients themselves will come to review their images and discuss directly with their radiologist.

## 3.2 Our Clinical Setup and How We Measured Its Value and Impact on Workflow

The LCC-embedded radiology reading room was established nearly a decade ago, within a conference room in the clinic, and consists of two diagnostic radiology workstations, staffed by an attending thoracic radiologist and a resident or fellow through typical workday hours (8 am to 5 pm), on a daily basis as part of routine clinical schedule. Attending radiologists rotate through this location as well as the main reading room. The radiologist assigned to the LCC, whenever not engaged in consultations, reads examinations from the same work lists on PACS and shares the workload in a relatively balanced fashion with three or four additional thoracic radiologists, who are located in the main hospital reading room.

> **The University of Pennsylvania and the LCC in numbers**
>
> - The thoracic imaging section is staffed by ten subspecialty trained thoracic radiologists, four or five of them simultaneously on clinical service every day.
> - Between 120 and 200 chest CTs and 300 and 500 chest radiographs daily.
> - At the LCC, 1 attending radiologist and 1 fellow/resident provide between 5 and 30 consultations every day to physicians and advanced practitioners (nurses, physician assistants).
> - The LCC practitioners see between 30 and 80 patients per day.

While our qualitative experience with the LCC model is that it improves patient care and strengthens relationships between radiologists and referring physicians, we performed a study to quantitate how referring physicians assess the value of having continued, unhindered access to a thoracic radiologist while they are seeing patients, and documented their perceptions about this service. In parallel, we assessed the frequency, duration, and number of consultations and how these impact radiologist's workflow.

In a recently published study (Mortani Barbosa and Novak 2018), we measured the utility and time commitment of our integrated thoracic radiologists in the multidisciplinary LCC with a consultancy log and a survey of referring physicians.

Over the course of 6 months, we measured the number, type, and duration of consultations in a consultancy log. We recorded 259 consultations over 44 clinical shifts (4 h each), in which 272 patients were discussed. Most consultations last between 2 and 5 min (75%), and in total consultations comprise approximately 10% of radiologist time, on average (though in busy days it can reach 25–30%).

Q3. How useful is it to have a real-time in-person consultation with a thoracic radiologist during clinic?

Q4. What percent of these consultations benefit patient care or add clinical value, over and above receiving the dictated report alone?

Q5. What percent of these consultations change management, over and above receiving the dictated report alone?

Q6. What do you find most valuable about embedded thoracic radiologists in the LC?

We sent the survey to all qualified LCC healthcare practitioners, and obtained a response rate of 86.4% (51 out of 59 eligible providers), indicating that the referring providers feel strongly about and value the presence of a constantly available thoracic radiologist in the LCC.

The vast majority of providers (90.2%, $n = 46$) interact with thoracic radiologists in the embedded reading room at the LCC clinic at least once a week, and all respondents at least once a month. This demonstrates that this is a highly sought-after service. Not only do most providers seek the opinion of our thoracic radiologists frequently, but they also praise the quality of the service they get.

---

**The most common reasons for consultation:**
- To clarify interpretation of imaging studies and diagnoses
- To assess for temporal changes
- In up to 25% of the times to discuss management options

---

In parallel, we ought to clarify the impact and value that we provide via a survey sent to the referring providers. The survey was comprised by the following questions:

Q1. How frequently do you review a case with a radiologist in the embedded LCC reading room?

Q2. How frequently do you review a case with a radiologist in the regular radiology reading room (main hospital)?

---

**Key Results of the Survey**
- **Overwhelming positive response from the referring providers:** unanimously rated the usefulness of this service as extremely high (90.2%) or high (9.8%).
- **Major positive impact on patient care/management:** 90.2% of providers believe that the consultations are beneficial in >60% of times; 51.0% think that these are beneficial in >80% of times; 86.2% of providers responded that their management changed because of the radiology consultation at least 50% of times.
- **What providers found most valuable:** rapid resolution of clinical questions or concerns (90.2%); deeper and higher level interaction with subspecialist chest radiologists (76.5%).

Multiple free-text comments were also entered, by 39.2% of respondents, including for example "This is an absolutely great program. Our radiology colleagues enable us to provide the best possible care to our patients. This service is EXTREMELY valuable to providing cutting edge, high quality care." Qualitative analysis of free-text comments (which were provided by 20/51 respondents, 39.2%) revealed that all except one of the comments were highly positive and indicated a high level of satisfaction and praise for the service we provide.

In summary, our research demonstrates that having a radiologist in the LCC-embedded reading room always available for real-time consultations is deemed extremely valuable by the referring clinicians, who enthusiastically endorse the value we provide to patient care through optimal, expedited diagnosis and management, and hold our radiologist and the consultative services we provide in high esteem. At the same time, consultations comprise a significant proportion of radiologist time, which existing payment models in the United States do not account for.

## 3.3 Conclusions and Implications for the Future of Radiology

Our experience in our integrated LCC reading room over the past 9 years has been extremely rewarding. The overwhelming positive response and praise from providers in the LCC is a testament to the perceived substantial value generated by the on-site presence of a radiologist consultant integrated within the clinic. However, the value of having a radiologist embedded in the LCC is not compensated in any form; moreover, the numerous daily consultations take a substantial amount of time from the radiologist, diverting him/her from RVU-producing activities, as the current fee-for-service RVU-centric payment model in the United States does not account for radiology consultative services. In other words, the radiologists are penalized, from a compensation standpoint, for providing a service that is highly valued and praised by the referring physicians, who enthusiastically endorse their benefit to patient care and management. Clearly, there is misalignment of incentives.

Several alternative payment models, such as value-based purchasing, explicitly account for performance and quality metrics to either increase or decrease compensation, and mandates for implementation of such models will effect major changes in the healthcare landscape. Other models such as bundled payments or capitation are also being considered. Another possibility is a division of revenue from the clinic operation between the frontline physicians and the consultant radiologists. Payment models are currently in a state of flux and it is impossible to forecast what exactly will happen within the next decades; nonetheless, radiology will have to proactively demonstrate the value it can provide to frontline healthcare providers, patients, and payers, in order to defend and increase our relevance in the future. For that purpose, we strongly believe that becoming a consultant, who is actively, constantly, and directly involved in all facets of patient care—beyond merely generating a text report for an imaging study—will be the salvation of our specialty. We must continue to expand our scope of practice beyond an isolated reading room to integrate ourselves within clinical practices, wherever it may be from the hospital wards to the subspecialty clinics, to ensure we are relevant, helpful, and valuable to patients and referring providers and therefore ensuring the very best and most cost-effective care for all patients.

**Radiologists do much more than just generating text reports:**
- We are expert diagnosticians.
- We ensure optimal and safe utilization of imaging equipment by designing and overseeing imaging acquisition protocols.
- We foster appropriate imaging utilization utilizing best available evidence.
- We educate providers about most cost-effective ways to diagnose and manage their patients utilizing imaging.
- We teach providers, from trainees to attending-level physicians, not only on imaging interpretation but also on complex diagnostic reasoning in challenging clinical settings.
- We provide consultations that impact patient diagnosis and management.
- We perform research that will change the future of medicine.

In the past, frontline physicians had to consult with radiologists primarily because they just did not have access to the images or reports on a timely fashion, but also because they thought that the consultations were positively impactful for their decision-making process. The difference is that nowadays, when we have nearly instantaneous access to images and very fast access to the reports (turnaround times were measured in weeks, rather than minutes, decades ago), we should strive to become consultants that will draw referring providers back to us, because the referring physicians want to directly discuss their patients with us, and not because they need to. And they would do it because they perceive that it is best for themselves and their patients, best for the quality of care they provide, best for expedite and accurate decision-making, and the most cost-effective approach to diagnosis and management.

## 4    Summary

We have reviewed two different practices of radiology consult, both in the field of thoracic imaging subspecialty: the German, in the Thoraxklinik University Heidelberg, comprising not just diagnostic but also interventional consultancy services for both the patients and providers, and the North American, at the University of Pennsylvania in Philadelphia, where referring providers have an extremely positive opinion of the value provided by this consultative service as we have seen through the results of the survey our published research.

Nevertheless, current payment models do not incentivize this arrangement, and we must actively strive to change these. In the era of precision medicine and patient-centered care, we believe that our work suggests a pathway not only to better delivery of care, communication, and coordination among teams of healthcare practitioners, but also increases quality of care and may enable a brighter future for radiology and the continued relevance of our specialty, in spite of multiple threats. Our vision is that the radiologist should be an active, visible, available, crucial member of the healthcare team, practicing in the core of a patient-centered model that is organized and oriented towards enabling maximum quality of care with minimal delays, redundancy, and bureaucratic obstacles, by providing his/her expertise on a real-time basis. The integrated radiology practice setup we proposed can be implemented in most mid- to large-size hospitals. The radiologist as a consultant is at the same time the future of our specialty and also a return to a past in which the interaction of radiologists and referring practitioners was the foundation of diagnosis and medical decision-making.

# References

Gunn AJ, Mangano MD, Choy G, Sahani DV (2015) Rethinking the role of the radiologist: enhancing visibility through both traditional and nontraditional reporting practices. Radiographics 35(2): 416–423

Heussel CP, Kauczor HU, Heussel G et al (1997) Early detection of pneumonia in febrile neutropenic patients: use of thin-section CT. AJR Am J Roentgenol 169(5):1347–1353

Jo HE, Glaspole IN, Levin KC et al (2016 Nov) Clinical impact of the interstitial lung disease multidisciplinary service. Respirology 21(8):1438–1444

Mangano MD, Bennett SE, Gunn AJ, Sahani DV, Choy G (2015) Creating a patient-centered radiology practice through the establishment of a diagnostic radiology consultation clinic. AJR Am J Roentgenol 205(1):95–99

Mortani Barbosa EJ Jr, Novak S (2018) The value of real-time thoracic radiology consulting in an Integrated Lung Center Clinic: bringing the radiologist to the Center of Multidisciplinary Health Care. J Thorac Imaging 33(4):260–265

# Value-Based Management of Incidental Findings

Sabine Weckbach and Oyunbileg von Stackelberg

## Contents

### Abstract

Radiological incidental findings (IFs) occur in research and diagnostic imaging. They are findings whose discovery is not intended. Due to a strong increase in high-tech imaging modalities the prevalence of IFs has risen. IFs regularly evoke discussions about accompanying ethical challenges. General principles to be considered in the management of IFs are responsibility for the well-being of the patient/study participant and of the society. In order to avoid overdiagnosis and overtherapy and generate a high value for patients, radiologists as well as clinicians need to know how to manage IFs. Over the last years, important guidelines ("white papers") for the handling of IFs have been published by different national and international imaging societies. Experiences from population-based research and measurement of value markers might trigger the further development and adaption of value-based guidelines.

## 1 Definition of Incidental Findings in Radiology

All findings could be called IFs when occurring in the context of medical diagnostics, potentially affecting the health of an individual and when not intended to be detected. However, it seems to be wrong to define an incidental finding only when

S. Weckbach (✉) · O. von Stackelberg
Diagnostic and Interventional Radiology,
University Hospital Heidelberg, Heidelberg, Germany
e-mail: Sabine.Weckbach@med.uni-heidelberg.de;
Oyunbileg.Stackelberg@med.uni-heidelberg.de

Med Radiol Diagn Imaging (2019)
https://doi.org/10.1007/174_2019_215, © Springer Nature Switzerland AG
Published Online: 02 July 2019

there is sufficient relevance for the health of a person. The concept of an incidental finding also includes marginal findings with no clinical relevance and false-positive findings (whose nature usually only becomes clear after further workup). IFs can occur in the context of research or while diagnostic methods are used to confirm or rule out the presence of a certain disease and also during follow-up examinations. Diagnostic findings that occur in the context of the doctor-patient relationship while searching for the cause of certain symptoms, but do not meet the doctor's expectations, are not IFs. The occurrence of an incidental finding, in this way, is not unexpected. Nowadays it is basic knowledge that the use of high-resolution imaging yields a relatively high number of findings that were not aimed at detecting. IFs should therefore be characterized as unintended findings whose discovery was not intended by a treating physician or medical researcher (Wolf et al. 2008).

In the relevant literature, the concept of IFs is, however, often used in a narrower sense. Incidental findings are characterized by three features:

1. They occur in participants during a scientific study.
2. They potentially affect the health of the concerned participant.
3. They are findings the discovery of which was not intended in the context of the study's aim.

Apart from research, an incidental finding can be described as a radiological finding not intentionally searched for, or an incidentally discovered mass or lesion, detected by an imaging modality, performed for an unrelated reason (Wolf et al. 2008; Schmücker 2012; Joerden et al. 2013).

Incidentally detected masses or tumorlike lesions are often called "incidentalomas," especially if they affect the adrenal glands (adrenal incidentaloma). It is important to understand that the term incidentaloma is not a diagnosis, but only a description of how the lesion was detected. Not uncommonly, the term is incorrectly used to denote a benign finding. In fact, the

term incidentaloma says nothing about the character or etiology of the lesion found.

> **Key Points**
> – Incidental findings occur in research and diagnostic imaging.
> – They can be described as radiological findings not intentionally searched for, or an incidentally discovered mass or lesion, detected by an imaging modality, performed for an unrelated reason.

## 2 Ethical Aspects of Incidental Findings

Incidental findings regularly evoke a discussion about ethical challenges that accompany them. They don't pose per se a critical ethical issue; they can be beneficial and lifesaving under certain circumstances. Under different circumstances though, such as when an incidental finding turns out to be a false positive, they can cause unnecessary follow-up or severe life-threatening complications (e.g., biopsy) and major distress (Schmidt et al. 2016). It is mainly the handling of IFs, then, that determines whether an incidental finding might be helpful or harmful, and therefore ethically critical or not (Erdmann 2015a, b; Fischer et al. 2015).

In December 2013, the Presidential Commission for the Study of Bioethical Issues (Bioethics Commission) released a report, *Anticipate and Communicate: Ethical Management of Incidental and Secondary Findings in the Clinical, Research, and Direct-to-Consumer Contexts* (Weiner 2014). The Bioethics Commission recommends that clinicians should have procedures in place including:

– Clear informed consent processes and communication strategies that convey the plan for managing IFs
– Use of tools to engage in shared decision-making with patients; strategies for effective communication about the risks associated with IFs and their follow-up

– Selective diagnostic testing to minimize the likelihood of IFs
– An awareness and understanding of existing clinical guidance for the management of incidental and secondary findings

## 3 General Principles to be Considered in the Management of Incidental Findings

- *Responsibility for the well-being of the patient/study participant*: A patient/study participant should be informed about health concerning IFs. This is in accordance with European and international ethical guidelines, e.g., Article 26 of the Additional Protocol to the Convention on Human Rights and Biomedicine, concerning Biomedical Research of the Council of Europe (Council of Europe 1999, 2007).
- *Responsibility for the well-being of the society*: The general population might be affected from undisclosed illnesses a participant might suffer from. This includes illnesses that might carry a risk for the patient/participant to cause a traffic accident. This is in accordance with Article 26 of the Convention for the Protection of Human Rights and Dignity of the Human Being with regard to the Application of Biology and Medicine: Convention on Human Rights and Biomedicine of the Council of Europe (Council of Europe 1999).

## 4 Frequency of Incidental Findings

Generally, IFs can occur in clinical imaging and in clinical research. The frequency with which they occur naturally differs depending on the application of technique, the defined field of view, the purpose of the examination, as well as the expertise of the person who interprets the images.

Since there has been a strong increase in the utilization and quality of high-tech imaging modalities as computed tomography (CT), magnetic

resonance (MR), and positron emission tomography (PET) imaging, IFs become increasingly prevalent. While whole-body MR scanning has become popular for large-scale population-based studies, the major cause for the detection of IFs in clinical imaging is CT scanning (Berlin 2011). In a recent retrospective study (based on radiology report review) of 1040 consecutive abdominal contrast-enhanced CT examinations (mean age 66 years) relevant IFs, i.e., findings leading to further imaging, clinical evaluation, or follow-up, were found in 19% (Sconfienza et al. 2015). There was an increase with patient age. The distribution among the involved organs was kidneys (14%), gallbladder (14%), lung (12%), uterus (10%), adrenal (10%), and vessels (10%). In total, 39 different types of relevant IFs were made on the 1040 contrast-enhanced abdominal CT examinations.

Welch has summarized the appearance of IFs as follows: 50% in the lungs on chest CTs, 23% in the kidneys, 15% in the liver on abdominal CTs, and 67% in the thyroid gland on ultrasound of the neck (Gilbert Welch et al. 2011). His comprehensive review of the radiologic literature disclosed that less than 4% of lung nodules and overall less than 1% of IFS elsewhere evolve into a lethal carcinoma.

As examples of IFs in research imaging, the overall prevalence of IFs on brain MRI examinations in the Rotterdam Study (Bos et al. 2016) was 9.5% (549 findings in 5800 participants; mean age 64.9 years). Of these, most common are meningiomas and cerebral aneurysms. In the study of health in Pommerania (SHIP) there were 1330 IFs of potential clinical relevance in 904 subjects (36.2%). The abdominal organs (6.8%), the urinary tract (6.8%), and the skeletal system (6.0%) were affected most often. More than 50% of findings were of an unclear nature (Hegenscheid et al. 2013).

> **Key Points**
> – A strong increase in the utilization and quality of high-tech imaging modalities has led to an increasing prevalence of IFs.
> – The major cause for IFs in clinical imaging is CT scanning.

## 5 Management of Incidental Findings in Research

Incidental findings in cohort studies is of course a rare subset of the whole IFS issue with only little effect on the healthcare system in contrast to the uncounted IFs in clinical imaging. Concerning value-based radiology, however, results from these cohort studies are very interesting and important in order to measure frequency and clinical relevance and set up appropriate guidelines and recommendations.

It is important to understand that there are different approaches concerning the management of IFs in different population-based imaging studies currently undertaken since so far no internationally obligatory guidelines exist. In this chapter, two quite different approaches to the management of IFs in the two largest population-based imaging studies currently undertaken in Europe are briefly depicted.

### 5.1 UK Biobank

The UK Biobank IF policy was developed following an extensive process which involved reviewing existing policies for the feedback of findings in UK Biobank participants, publishing evidence and guidance on IFs, receiving external legal advice on the scope of the duty of care, and consulting with the independent UK Biobank Ethics and Governance Council, UK Biobank's major funders (Wellcome Trust and Medical Research Council), and with the Royal College of Radiologists and the Society and College of Radiographers. UK Biobank also consulted with relevant experts to explore the legal and ethical factors which were applicable to the development of the IF policy.

The UK Biobank IF protocol was developed from first principles as a pragmatic protocol that could be implemented on a large scale with the objective of striking the optimum balance of most net benefit and least net harm to 100,000 largely asymptomatic participants (Sudlow et al. 2015). Under this protocol, participants only receive feedback in specific, lim-ited circumstances: when a radiographer identifies a potentially serious incidental finding during the acquisition or quality assessment of images during the imaging visit, and when a radiologist subsequently confirms the presence of a potentially serious IF. UK Biobank defines a potentially serious imaging incidental finding as "a finding which indicates the possibility of a condition which, if confirmed, would carry a real prospect of seriously threatening life span, or of having a substantial impact on major body functions or quality of life" (Sudlow et al. 2015).

### 5.2 German National Cohort (GNC)

The German National Cohort is a long-term, multicenter, population-based cohort study currently undertaken in Germany with the goal of investigating the development of common chronic diseases. As part of this investigation, 30,000 out of the total of 200,000 participants are being subjected to a whole-body 3-Tesla MR imaging without contrast agents. To help with the implementation of national and international ethical guidelines a system was developed to classify and report IFs that might be detected on imaging and possibly pose a risk to the participant's health. This system focuses on guiding radiologists in the decision of reporting or not reporting a finding in an attempt to balance the risk of over- and underreporting, and thus to minimize false positives and false negatives. The cornerstone of that process is a list specifying findings and separating them into report-worthy and not-report-worthy. For defining IFs, study-specific limitations and confounders had to be taken into account. Within this list, report-worthy IFs were classified into acutely relevant and non-acutely relevant findings. Acutely relevant findings were defined as suspected disease for which the participant should receive immediate clinical care. Examples include possible stroke, pneumothorax, and aortic dissection. These findings have to be reported in a timely manner not only for the benefit of the participant but also to avoid danger to the public, for example, from causing a traffic accident. Non-acutely relevant findings are reported within 10 working days.

## 6 Management of Incidental Findings in Clinical Imaging

Before IFs even arise, radiologists have to decide about the appropriate imaging method: Is it possible to reduce IFs by choosing a different imaging method? When an incidental finding is then detected, we have to be aware that the description of an unexpected finding can trigger additional medical care including unnecessary tests, other diagnostic procedures, and treatments which in some cases may pose an additional risk to the patient and generate high costs or could be life-saving in other cases.

We have to focus on value as well as outcomes and therefore ask the following questions:

1. Which IFs do we address?
2. How do we address IFs?
3. Do we need follow-up imaging or other diagnostic procedures?
4. Can undesirable consequences be avoided (Lumbreras et al. 2010)?

In order to especially avoid overdiagnosis and overtherapy and generate a high value for patients, radiologists as well as clinicians need to know how to deal with unexpected findings.

Nowadays, it is common sense that IFs should be categorized into

– Actionable (urgently/non-urgently)
– Non-actionable

For further and detailed guidance, there have been several important guidelines published by different national and international imaging societies ("white papers") for the handling of IFs in a daily clinical care over the last years. Since 2010 the ACR Incidental Findings Committee has published several white papers on management of IFs on abdominal and pelvic CT and MRI, adrenal, vascular, splenic, nodal, gallbladder, biliary, thyroid, liver, renal and adrenal masses, pancreatic cyst, as well as pituitary findings and mediastinal and cardiovascular findings on thoracic CT (Berland et al. 2010; Gore et al. 2017; Heller et al. 2013; Herts et al. 2018; Khosa et al. 2013; Mayo-Smith et al. 2017; Megibow et al. 2017; Patel et al. 2013; Sebastian et al. 2013; Munden et al. 2018; Hoang et al. 2015, 2018; Berland 2013).

For example, the prevalence of noncalcified lung nodules on multi-detector CT (MDCT) has been reported as 33% (range 17–53%) and 13% (range 2–24%), in a screening and non-screening study population, respectively (Callister et al. 2015). However, the prevalence of malignancy in nodules measuring <5 mm is very low, ranging between 0% and 1% (Horeweg et al. 2014). Since the increase in the detection rate of small pulmonary nodules, the clinical significance of these findings represents a new challenge, and the optimal management of each case becomes pivotal and should be conducted according to the clinical setting (Larici et al. 2017). In 2017 the Fleischner Society has published a revised guideline for management of incidental pulmonary nodules. In this guideline the minimum threshold size for routine follow-up has been increased, and recommended follow-up intervals are now given as a range rather than as a precise time period to give radiologists, clinicians, and patients greater discretion to accommodate individual risk factors and preferences (MacMahon et al. 2017). Most of the guidelines however target radiologist and the recommendations assume a level of radiological expertise (O'Sullivan et al. 2018). Clinicians, particularly primary care physicians, are unsure which incidentalomas require urgent further investigation, nor are they sure which incidentalomas are likely to be benign (Sexton 2014). Systematic reviews on prevalence and malignancy of incidentalomas, such as the review by O'Sullivan et al., aid clinicians and patients to weigh up the pros and cons of requesting imaging scans and will help with management decisions after an incidentaloma diagnosis (O'Sullivan et al. 2018).

Over the last years, the awareness for value-based healthcare has risen. The Image Wisely® and Image Gently® initiatives (https://qpp.cms. gov/mips/explore-measures/quality-measures? py=2018&specialtyMeasureSet=Diagnostic%20 Radiology) have the goal to address radiation safety concerns and to decrease the exposure to the patient as well as to eliminate unnecessary procedures. It is important that radiologists are available for referring physicians to collaborate and advise how to handle IFs. The other aspect, which is extremely important, is to put always the patient at the center of care. A team-based approach with the referring doctor, the radiologist, the patient, and the administration will improve healthcare and continue to provide value.

Recently, the American Medical Association has started to publish criteria for value markers and to specify how value is measured referring also to IFs (https://qpp.cms.gov/mips/explore-measures/quality-measures?py=2018&specialty MeasureSet=Diagnostic%20Radiology). This approach is new and the results have to be closely watched for the development and adaption of value-based guidelines in the future.

---

**Key Points**

- Overdiagnosis and overtherapy of IFs have to be avoided.
- IFs should be categorized into action-able (urgently/non-urgently) and non-actionable.
- Radiologists and clinicians need to know how to manage IFs.
- Detailed guidance is provided by several important guidelines published by different national and international imaging societies ("white papers).
- A team-based approach with the referring physician, the radiologist, and the patient with the patient in the center of care will lead to a successful, value-based management of IFs.

# References

Berland LL (2013) Overview of white papers of the ACR incidental findings committee ii on adnexal, vascular, splenic, nodal, gallbladder, and biliary findings. J Am Coll Radiol 10(9):672–674

Berland LL, Silverman SG, Gore RM, Mayo-Smith WW, Megibow AJ, Yee J, Brink JA, Baker ME, Federle MP, Foley WD et al (2010) Managing incidental findings on abdominal CT: white paper of the ACR incidental findings committee. J Am Coll Radiol 7(10):754–773

Berlin L (2011) The incidentaloma: a medicolegal dilemma. Radiol Clin N Am 49(2):245–255

Bos D, Poels MM, Adams HH, Akoudad S, Cremers LG, Zonneveld HI, Hoogendam YY, Verhaaren BF, Verlinden VJ, Verbruggen JG et al (2016) Prevalence, clinical management, and natural course of incidental findings on brain MR images: the population-based Rotterdam scan study. Radiology 281(2):507–515

Callister ME, Baldwin DR, Akram AR, Barnard S, Cane P, Draffan J, Franks K, Gleeson F, Graham R, Malhotra P et al (2015) British Thoracic Society guidelines for the investigation and management of pulmonary nodules. Thorax 70(Suppl 2):ii1–ii54

Council of Europe (1999) Convention for the protection of human rights and dignity of the human being with regard to the application of biology and medicine: convention on human rights and biomedicine. Council of Europe, Strasbourg, France

Council of Europe (2007) Additional Protocol to the Convention on Human Rights and Biomedicine, concerning Biomedical Research. Council of Europe Steering Committee on Bioethics, Strasbourg, France

Erdmann P (2015a) Zufallsbefunde aus bildgebenden Verfahren in populationsbasierter Forschung. Mentis, Münster

Erdmann P (2015b) Handling incidental findings from imaging within IM related research—results from an empirical-ethical study. In: Fischer T, Langanke M, Marschall P, Michl S (eds) Individualized medicine: ethical, economical and historical perspectives. Springer International Publishing, Cham, pp 231–250

Fischer T, Langanke M, Marschall P, Michl S (2015) Individualized medicine. Ethical, economical and historical perspectives. Springer, Heidelberg, pp 231–250

Gilbert Welch H, Schwartz LM, Woloshin S (2011) Overdiagnosed: making people sick in the pursuit of health. Beacon Press, Boston, MA

Gore RM, Pickhardt PJ, Mortele KJ, Fishman EK, Horowitz JM, Fimmel CJ, Talamonti MS, Berland LL, Pandharipande PV (2017) Management of incidental liver lesions on CT: a white paper of the ACR incidental findings committee. J Am Coll Radiol 14(11):1429–1437

Hegenscheid K, Seipel R, Schmidt CO, Volzke H, Kuhn JP, Biffar R, Kroemer HK, Hosten N, Puls R (2013) Potentially relevant incidental findings on research whole-body MRI in the general adult population: frequencies and management. Eur Radiol 23(3):816–826

Heller MT, Harisinghani M, Neitlich JD, Yeghiayan P, Berland LL (2013) Managing incidental findings on abdominal and pelvic CT and MRI, part 3: white paper of the ACR incidental findings committee II on splenic and nodal findings. J Am Coll Radiol 10(11):833–839

Herts BR, Silverman SG, Hindman NM, Uzzo RG, Hartman RP, Israel GM, Baumgarten DA, Berland LL, Pandharipande PV (2018) Management of the incidental renal mass on CT: a white paper of the ACR incidental findings committee. J Am Coll Radiol 15(2):264–273

Hoang JK, Langer JE, Middleton WD, Wu CC, Hammers LW, Cronan JJ, Tessler FN, Grant EG, Berland LL (2015) Managing incidental thyroid nodules detected on imaging: white paper of the ACR incidental thyroid findings committee. J Am Coll Radiol 12(2):143–150

Hoang JK, Hoffman AR, Gonzalez RG, Wintermark M, Glenn BJ, Pandharipande PV, Berland LL, Seidenwurm DJ (2018) Management of incidental pituitary findings on CT, MRI, and (18)F-Fluorodeoxyglucose PET: a white paper of the ACR incidental findings committee. J Am Coll Radiol 15(7):966–972

Horeweg N, van Rosmalen J, Heuvelmans MA, van der Aalst CM, Vliegenthart R, Scholten ET, ten Haaf K, Nackaerts K, Lammers JW, Weenink C et al (2014) Lung cancer probability in patients with CT-detected pulmonary nodules: a prespecified analysis of data from the NELSON trial of low-dose CT screening. Lancet Oncol 15(12):1332–1341

https://qpp.cms.gov/mips/explore-measures/quality-measures?py=2018&specialtyMeasureSet=Diagnostic%20Radiology

Joerden JC, Hilgendorf E, Thiele F (2013) Menschenwürde und Medizin. Duncker & Humblot, Berlin

Khosa F, Krinsky G, Macari M, Yucel EK, Berland LL (2013) Managing incidental findings on abdominal and pelvic CT and MRI, part 2: white paper of the ACR incidental findings committee II on vascular findings. J Am Coll Radiol 10(10):789–794

Larici AR, Farchione A, Franchi P, Ciliberto M, Cicchetti G, Calandriello L, Del Ciello A, Bonomo L (2017) Lung nodules: size still matters. Eur Respir Rev 26(146)

Lumbreras B, Donat L, Hernandez-Aguado I (2010) Incidental findings in imaging diagnostic tests: a systematic review. Br J Radiol 83(988):276–289

MacMahon H, Naidich DP, Goo JM, Lee KS, Leung ANC, Mayo JR, Mehta AC, Ohno Y, Powell CA, Prokop M et al (2017) Guidelines for management of incidental pulmonary nodules detected on CT images: from the Fleischner Society 2017. Radiology 284(1):228–243

Mayo-Smith WW, Song JH, Boland GL, Francis IR, Israel GM, Mazzaglia PJ, Berland LL, Pandharipande PV (2017) Management of incidental adrenal masses: a white paper of the ACR incidental findings committee. J Am Coll Radiol 14(8):1038–1044

Megibow AJ, Baker ME, Morgan DE, Kamel IR, Sahani DV, Newman E, Brugge WR, Berland LL, Pandharipande PV (2017) Management of incidental pancreatic cysts: a white paper of the ACR incidental findings committee. J Am Coll Radiol 14(7):911–923

Munden RF, Carter BW, Chiles C, MacMahon H, Black WC, Ko JP, McAdams HP, Rossi SE, Leung AN, Boiselle PM et al (2018) Managing incidental findings on thoracic CT: mediastinal and cardiovascular findings. A white paper of the ACR incidental findings committee. J Am Coll Radiol 15(8):1087–1096

O'Sullivan JW, Muntinga T, Grigg S, Ioannidis JPA (2018) Prevalence and outcomes of incidental imaging findings: umbrella review. BMJ 361:k2387

Patel MD, Ascher SM, Paspulati RM, Shanbhogue AK, Siegelman ES, Stein MW, Berland LL (2013) Managing incidental findings on abdominal and pelvic CT and MRI, part 1: white paper of the ACR incidental findings committee II on adnexal findings. J Am Coll Radiol 10(9):675–681

Schmidt CO, Sierocinski E, Hegenscheid K, Baumeister SE, Grabe HJ, Volzke H (2016) Impact of whole-body MRI in a general population study. Eur J Epidemiol 31(1):31–39

Schmücker R (2012) Zufallsbefunde – was gebietet die Menschenwürde? In: Preprints and working papers of the centre for advanced study in bioethics. WWU, Munster

Sconfienza LM, Mauri G, Muzzupappa C, Poloni A, Bandirali M, Esseridou A, Tritella S, Secchi F, Di Leo G, Sardanelli F (2015) Relevant incidental findings at abdominal multi-detector contrast-enhanced computed tomography: a collateral screening? World J Radiol 7(10):350–356

Sebastian S, Araujo C, Neitlich JD, Berland LL (2013) Managing incidental findings on abdominal and pelvic CT and MRI, part 4: white paper of the ACR incidental findings committee II on gallbladder and biliary findings. J Am Coll Radiol 10(12):953–956

Sexton SM (2014) How should we manage incidentalomas? Am Fam Physician 90(11):758–759

Sudlow C, Gallacher J, Allen N, Beral V, Burton P, Danesh J, Downey P, Elliott P, Green J, Landray M et al (2015) UK Biobank: an open access resource for identifying the causes of a wide range of complex diseases of middle and old age. PLoS Med 12(3):e1001779

Weiner C (2014) Anticipate and communicate: Ethical management of incidental and secondary findings in the clinical, research, and direct-to-consumer contexts (December 2013 report of the presidential commission for the study of bioethical issues). Am J Epidemiol 180(6):562–564

Wolf SM, Lawrenz FP, Nelson CA, Kahn JP, Cho MK, Clayton EW, Fletcher JG, Georgieff MK, Hammerschmidt D, Hudson K et al (2008) Managing incidental findings in human subjects research: analysis and recommendations. J Law Med Ethics 36(2):219–248, 211

# The Value in Artificial Intelligence

Ramandeep Singh, Fatemeh Homayounieh,
Rachel Vining, Subba R. Digumarthy,
and Mannudeep K. Kalra

## Contents

## Abstract

Past 5 years have seen burgeoning applications of machine learning (ML) in diverse radiological domains including thoracic radiology, neuroimaging, abdominal imaging, musculoskeletal imaging, and breast imaging. Deep learning technologies have been applied to improve image resolution at ultralow radiation dose. Publications abound on ML in chest CT have focused on detection and characterization of pulmonary nodules, as well as for rib and spine straightening and labeling, vessel segmentation, and estimation of CT fractional flow reserve. ML has also been applied for detecting lines, tubes, pneumothorax, pleural effusions, cardiomegaly, and pneumonia, on chest radiographs. Applications of ML in cerebral hemorrhage detection and prediction of stroke outcomes, appendicitis and renal colic prediction, hand bone age calculation or rib unfolding for fracture detection, and characterization of breast macro-calcifications and masses are also shown. We review fundamentals, applications, and limitations of machine learning in thoracic radiology, neuroimaging, abdominal imaging, musculoskeletal imaging, and breast imaging.

R. Singh · F. Homayounieh · S. R. Digumarthy
M. K. Kalra (✉)
Division of Thoracic Imaging,
Massachusetts General Hospital, Boston, MA, USA

Harvard Medical School, Boston, MA, USA
e-mail: mkalra@mgh.harvard.edu

R. Vining
Division of Thoracic Imaging,
Massachusetts General Hospital, Boston, MA, USA

Med Radiol Diagn Imaging (2019)
https://doi.org/10.1007/174_2018_193, © Springer Nature Switzerland AG
Published Online: 19 February 2019

# 1    Introduction

Artificial intelligence (AI), a term used for computers with cognitive functions akin to human intelligence, incorporates learning by perception decision-making for solving issues. Machine learning (ML) refers to the ability of computers to learn with human-devised algorithms as well as to improve from experience without being explicitly programmed (Erickson et al. 2017).

Alan Turing introduced the concept of machine learning in the seminal paper on "Computing machinery and intelligence" in 1950. He described the "Turing test" to determine if a computer has intelligence. In the test, a judge types questions for the two entities—a person and a computer—and then deciphers responses for human and computer identities. If the judge is wrong, the computer passes the Turing test and is deemed as intelligent. Almost 70 years later, a reversed form of Turing test is still used on the Internet, known as the CAPTCHA test, to determine whether the user is a human or a computer.

> **Key Points**
> – **Artificial intelligence:** is a subspecialty of computer science devoted to creating systems to perform tasks that commonly require human intelligence.
> – **Machine learning:** is a subfield of AI, referring to the ability of computers to learn with human-devised algorithms, as well as to improve from experience, without being explicitly programmed.

The credit for coining the term "computer-aided diagnosis (CAD)" in the year 1975 goes to a remarkable radiologist, Gwilym S. Lodwick, who introduced application for image modeling, and computer-aided diagnosis for interpreting bone tumors on radiographs. Traditionally, CAD systems are classified as computer-aided detection (CADe) and computer-aided diagnosis (CADx). CADe localizes lesions, and CADx characterizes them (Firmino et al. 2016). Computer-aided detection/diagnosis (CAD) is based on image processing and interpretation using a large amount of information. A complex pattern recognition uses AI and computer vision. CAD server analyzes image data in a sequential manner for preprocessing noise and artifacts, and segmentation for differentiating anatomical structures and regions of interest for compactness and grey value. Finally, it uses different algorithms for classification/character analysis. The first report on CAD in imaging was published in 1963, and described the role of chest radiographs in predicting prognosis of primary lung cancer (Lodwick et al. 1963). The radiographic findings were converted into numerical codes for lesion location, size, shape, contour, density, and calcification, and then interpreted for malignancy by a computer. Limitations of CAD without ML included high false-positive rates which prolonged interpretation times, and at times led to additional biopsies (Firmino et al. 2016).

> **Key Points**
> – **CAD:** introduced by Gwilym S. Lodwick in 1975, a radiologist who was nominated for Nobel Prize, has serious limitations without machine learning.

In radiology, ML algorithms use radiological images, reports, and annotations as training datasets to generate a model with learning methods that can be either unsupervised or supervised.

The input and output statistical probabilities are termed as nodes with included numeric weights known as hyperparameters. If the output data ensemble continuous values they denote a regression. The output data with categorized value are termed as classification (Chartrand et al. 2017). Training data are forward fed into a computation system, and then backpropagated over several cycles to form a

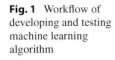

**Fig. 1** Workflow of
developing and testing
machine learning
algorithm

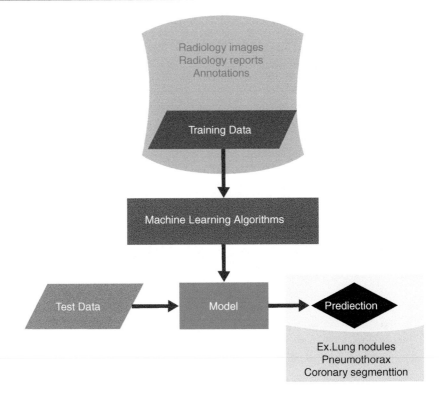

desirable model. Test data are then employed to predict response of the model for trained radiological findings such as lung nodule, pneumothorax, and coronary segmentation (Fig. 1). Repeat cycles of training and testing help optimize the algorithm, which can then be subjected to validation data.

To address lack of well-curated labeled data, a specific type of ML, representation learning (RL), has been introduced. This subtype of ML utilizes a self-learning approach to learn classifying features rather than hand-drafted features.

Deep learning (DL), a subtype of RL, involves learning with multilayered data representations instead of specifically devised algorithms. This technique employs hierarchal organization of layers of different data computational stages, for learning features and classification of patterns, like the human brain. Learning higher abstractions with multiple data representations enables the computer to perform image analyses. This is made possible by an architectural organization of artificial neural networks (Chartrand et al. 2017).

**Key Points**
- **Unsupervised machine learning:** employs unlabeled input data to describe a function with an elucidation of hidden structures.
- **Supervised machine learning:** incorporates input training data in a computational network that works in hidden layers to yield output data.
- **Representation learning:** a type of ML utilizing a self-learning approach to learn classifying features, replacing manual feature engineering.
- **Deep learning:** a subtype of RL involving learning with multilayered data, similar to human brain, and where the learned features are compositional or hierarchical.

Artificial neural networks (ANN) are computer systems that learn without being trained in a specific programmed manner. This learning process is akin to biological neural networks, with basic units of artificial neurons or nodes (Chartrand et al. 2017).

**Key Points**
- **Deep neural networks (DNN):** a subset of ANN having a complex architecture with nonlinear data flow in multiple stacked layers from input to output (Suk and Shen 2013). The first layer is the input data, intermediate layers are hidden layers for processing, and the last layer is output as classified results.
- **Convolutional neural network (CNN):** a type of DNN performing image analysis. It transfers each feature finder over each image part in a convolutional pattern and is not affected by the image distortions. CNN need lesser preprocessing as compared to other ML algorithms (Hua et al. 2015).
- **Deep belief network (DBN):** a type of CNN using a configuration of unsupervised network layers with hidden layers in each network. DBN can be trained to facilitate a fast, efficient training process (Hinton et al. 2006).
- **Fully convolutional networks (FCN):** process images in one forward pass and segment the input images pixel-wise. FCN import a pre-trained model to expedite transfer learning independent of dataset size (Lee et al. 2017a).

## 2 ML Applications in Thoracic Radiology: Chest Radiography

Chest radiographs are the most frequently performed imaging procedure, with volume far exceeding CT. Often chest radiographs are the initial and the only imaging examination, such as in remote areas or underdeveloped countries, where ML can help physicians with image interpretation and provide valuable information given the lack of radiological expertise.

### 2.1 Lung Nodules

CNN algorithms have been assessed for nodule detection on chest radiographs based on their size, shape, texture, and location (Wang et al. 2017a). Recent studies have demonstrated that ML-based commercial software (RapidScreen, Riverain Inc.) for evaluation of pulmonary nodules on chest radiograph was associated with a 23% increase in detection of 9–14 mm nodules on chest radiographs (Riverain 2004). Another study found that ML-based CAD system detected 40/81 (49.4%) of missed malignant nodules on chest radiographs (Kligerman et al. 2013).

Most ML methods use either a single hand-crafted feature or a single DL algorithm. A fusion method of DNN for lung nodule detection has been proposed with three modules: rib suppression to remove ribs, lung segmentation by active shape model, and retrieval of pulmonary nodules by generalized Laplacian of Gaussian method. This is followed by feature extraction based on parameters such as nodule geometry, intensity, and contrast. The single hand-crafted feature models have low sensitivity of 62% and false-positive rate (1.45 nodules per radiographs) but a high specificity of 95% (Wang et al. 2017a). The single DL method had 66% sensitivity, 96% specificity, and 1.3 false positive rate, whereas the fusion method of DNN had 69% sensitivity, 96% specificity, and the lowest false-positive rate of 1.19 per radiograph (Wang et al. 2017a).

### 2.2 Pulmonary Tuberculosis

Although chest radiography is the primary screening method for workup and follow-up of suspected and proven pulmonary tuberculosis, relative deficiency of trained manpower for accurate image-based recognition of pertinent findings has been cited as the reason for a suboptimal yield of World Health Organization's (WHO) fight against the disease (Melendez et al. 2016; Hoog et al. 2011). ML algorithms have been proposed to improve detection of pulmonary tuberculosis on chest radiographs.

Recent studies on dedicated CAD software (CADT4) which combines texture abnormality with shape detection of pulmonary tuberculosis on chest radiography reported an area under the curve (AUC) that ranged from 0.71 to 0.84 (Pande et al. 2016; Maduskar et al. 2013). Lung segmentation, texture, and feature extraction followed by classification with support vector machine (SVM) achieved an AUC of 0.87–0.90 (Jaeger et al. 2014). Hwang et al. have reported further improvement in accuracy (AUC between 0.88 and 0.96) for detecting pulmonary findings related to tuberculosis using a deep CNN-based ML algorithm (Hwang et al. 2016). In another study of 1007 frontal chest radiographs, using two deep CNNs—AlexNet and GoogLeNet—to classify radiographs as healthy or suggestive of pulmonary tuberculosis, the pre-trained models had the highest accuracy (AUC 0.99) (Lakhani and Sundaram 2017).

## 2.3    Pneumoconiosis

Presenting symptoms and chest radiograph findings are essential for diagnosis of pneumoconiosis. Chest radiographs are compared to International Labor Organization (ILO) standardized digital radiograph, for classification of radiographic abnormalities into four categories (0, I, II, and III). The progression from 0 to III correlates with increasing disease severity. Although standardized, the method lacks specificity for etiopathological condition of pneumoconiosis, and is ambiguous in classifying categories I and II as pneumoconiosis. These limitations offer an opportunity for ML to improve the diagnostic accuracy of chest radiographs for patients with suspected or known pneumoconiosis (Zhu et al. 2014).

Early CAD systems used texture analyses based on gray-level histogram co-occurrence matrix and geometric pattern feature analysis (Zhu et al. 2014; Yu et al. 2011). Evaluation with gray-level co-occurrence matrix-based features yielded a 95% accuracy for correct categorization of radiographic findings (Xu et al. 2010). SVM trained with texture features from healthy and pneumoconiosis patients had a 92.9% accuracy (AUC 0.974) for classification of chest radiographs in patients with pneumoconiosis (Zhu et al. 2014).

## 2.4    Pneumothorax Detection

New, increased, and tension pneumothoraces on chest radiographs are critical findings which require immediate interpretation, and communication with the healthcare providers. ML algorithms have been applied to expedite detection of pneumothorax on chest radiographs (AI 2017). A recent study of 644 chest radiographs with 311 radiographs positive for large pneumothorax reported that ML models [trained and untrained versions of AlexNet, GoogLeNet (Inception V1), and ResNet 34] had 94% sensitivity and 88% specificity for detection of pneumothorax on chest (AI 2017).

## 2.5    Position of the Peripherally Inserted Central Catheters (PICC)

Although there are now techniques to confirm the position of the PICC without radiographs, chest radiographs are still commonly used to confirm their position before use. Recently, ML application with patch-based approach has been applied to image interpretation with contrast-limited adaptive histogram equalization (CLAHE) to achieve consistent image contrast (Lee et al. 2017a). Post-processing removes bone edges and other high-density opacities to generate a final image with superimposed PICC line and tip location. The mean predicted location of the PICC tip from the ground truth was about 3 mm with a standard deviation of 2 mm (Lee et al. 2017a).

## 3    ML Applications in Thoracic Radiology: Chest CT

Several commercial ML applications in CT imaging have recently become available. Some modern MDCT scanners (Siemens Healthineers) now use ML to automatically acquire planning radiographs based on specified CT protocol. Furthermore, for cardiac CT applications, these ML algorithms can identify and insert a region of interest in the ascending thoracic aorta for bolus tracking or timing contrast bolus (Lee et al. 2017b). The United States Food and Drug Administration (FDA) approved chest CT interpretation (RAdLogics Virtual Resident) algorithm employing ML to analyze chest CT for specific imaging findings, and to insert these findings into the radiology reports. Although the algorithm cannot assess all abnormalities, it can detect and quantify pleural effusion or pneumothorax, detect and localize pulmonary opacities, and obtain dimension of thoracic aorta.

## 3.1 Pulmonary Nodules on CT

The earliest reported methods for lung nodule characterization entailed analysis of geometric features of pulmonary nodules based on multiple gray-level thresholds (Giger et al. 1994). These were supplanted with object-based deformation procedures, morphological analysis, and model-based techniques (Armato et al. 2003). Elimination of blood vessels and calcifications in

lung nodules using AI can enhance the sensitivity and specificity to 100% and 93%, respectively (Manikandan and Bharathi 2016).

ML-based vessel suppression algorithm (Riverain's ClearRead CT Vessel Suppress) claims a 0.58 false-positive rate per CT, and to improve the lung cancer detection from 0.633 without vessel suppression to 0.773 with vessel suppression algorithm (Figs. 2 and 3).

Initial CADe system for detection of pulmonary nodules had a low sensitivity (70%) with high false-positive rate of 9.6 nodules per chest CT (Armato et al. 1999), although Messay et al. reported recently (2010) much better sensitivity (about 83%) for lung nodule detection with only three false-positive lesions per chest CT (Messay et al. 2010). Also, early studies (2003) with neural networks by Suzuki et al. have reported a classification sensitivity of 93% and 4.8 false-positive nodules per CT (Suzuki et al. 2003).

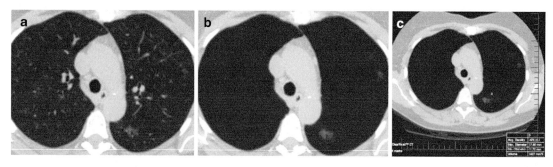

**Fig. 2** Compared to baseline CT image (**a**), subtraction of vessels with ML (ClearRead CT, Riverain Inc.), (**b**) makes it easy to classify the left lower lobe nodule as pure glass-ground nodule instead of part-solid. Estimated dimensions of same nodule with automatic detection (**c**)

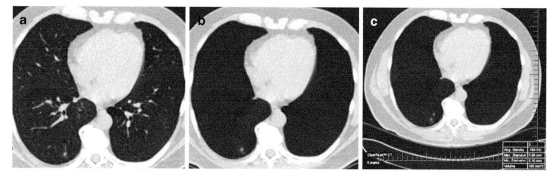

**Fig. 3** ML-assisted subtraction of vessels (ClearRead CT, Riverain Inc.) can help detect and accentuate the solid component on chest CT (**b**) and characterize the nodule in right lower lobe as a part-solid nodule, similar to its appearance on unprocessed image (**a**). The ML-based detection algorithm (**c**) measures only the solid component of nodule

## 3.2  Radiomics in Lung Cancer

Studies have demonstrated that radiomic features can help differentiate benign from malignant pulmonary nodules, and predict different mutations associated with lung cancer (Gillies et al. 2016; Lambin et al. 2012; Hawkins et al. 2016; Lee et al. 2014; Maldonado et al. 2013). Hawkins et al. investigated 23 radiomics features to predict malignant potential of lung nodules in the National Lung Screening Trial (NLST) CT database, and reported accuracies of 80% (AUC 0.83) for chest CT at 1 year, and 79% (AUC 0.75) at 2 years (Lambin et al. 2012). For part-solid nodules, in comparison to clinical and CT features alone, combination of radiomics improved the AUC from 79 to 93% for benign versus malignant etiologies (Hawkins et al. 2016). Several hundred radiomic features can be obtained from analysis of a single region of interest, which implies that applications and integration of radiomics into clinical workflow will require some form of ML algorithms.

Radiomics have been applied for evaluation of different sets of mutations associated with lung cancer; the information is helpful in formulating targeted pharmacotherapy. Previous studies on prediction of mutations in 353 patients using ML-based application of radiomic signatures for EGFR and KRAS mutations have yielded promising results (Maldonado et al. 2013). Radiomics could differentiate EGFR+ and EGFR− cases of lung cancer (AUC 0.69). Predictive radiomic signatures to differentiate EGFR+ and KRAS+ lung cancer had 87% specificity and 79% accuracy (0.80 AUC) (Rios Velazquez et al. 2017).

## 3.3  Vascular Applications

ML algorithms have been applied in commercially available vascular post-processing software for anatomical labeling of major blood vessels on CT images as well as in automatic extraction of curved planar reformats (CPR) along vessel centerline and short-axis views for luminal assessment (Fig. 4). Available ML applications aid in automatic measurement of thoracic and abdominal aortic aneurysms as well as in rapid measurement for transcutaneous aortic valve replacement (TAVR) planning. The three components of these algorithms are labeling of major vessels, measurement of diameters based on vessel area/perimeter, and generation of direct CPR with short-axis display.

For coronary CT angiography, ML has been applied for automatic segmentation and CPR of coronary arterial tree with labeling of main coronary arteries, major branches, and saphenous vein grafts. For ECG-gated cardiac CT, ML has been applied in auto-segmentation of ventricles, auto-calculation of global and local ventricular function, and display of myocardial first-pass perfusion defects.

Recent studies have validated use of fractional flow reserve (FFR) to assess hemodynamic significance of coronary stenosis on ECG-gated coronary CT angiogram (Rios Velazquez et al. 2017). However, manually intensive post-processing of CT data required several hours, and thus limited application of CT FFR. Recently, Itu et al. have reported that ML-assisted calculation of FFR on coronary CT angiogram had 83% accuracy with 2.4-s processing time, compared to 196 s with conventional FFR calculation (Rios Velazquez et al. 2017).

---

**Key Points**

**Main current applications of ML in thoracic radiology—*Pulmonary pathologies***

- Pulmonary nodule detection and characterization
- Pulmonary opacities: Pulmonary tuberculosis
  – Pneumoconiosis
- AI-based radiomics in lung cancer

**Main current applications of ML in thoracic radiology—*Extrapulmonary pathologies***

- Pneumothorax detection
- Lines and tubes on chest radiograph

- **Cardiac applications:** FFR calculation in coronary CT angiography
  - Segmentation of coronary arteries on CT
- **Vascular applications:** Automatic segmentation and display of aorta and its branches
  - Automatic recognition of vascular landmarks and branches
- **Bone applications:** Rib straightening and labeling
  - Spine straightening and vertebral body labeling

# 4    ML Applications in Neuroimaging

Main ML applications in brain have focused on detection of brain hemorrhage on CT, automatic labeling of the vertebral level on CT and MR images, and segmentation of various anatomic parts of the brain on MR. ML can also help create study protocols based on exam indication and clinical profiling for individual patient, particularly for brain and body MR examinations (Itu et al. 2016; Rothenberg et al. 2016). Anatomic MR can be reconstructed using sparse raw data from the scanner to decrease the acquisition time by more than 50% (Sohn et al. 2017; Hammernik

**Fig. 4** ML-assisted vascular CT application (SyngoVia, Siemens) enables automatic labeling, multiplanar display, and measurement of abdominal aorta and its branches

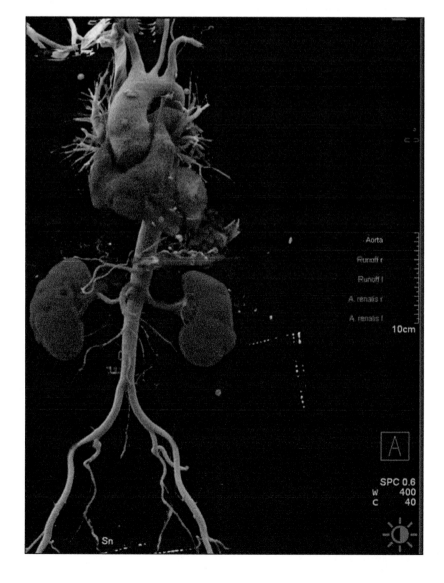

et al. 2017). SVM based ML can aid in detection of temporal lobe epilepsy on quantitative MR imaging (Golkov et al. 2016). MRI in scenarios like stroke or cerebral hemorrhage needs rapid acquisition and reporting, a problem that can be solved with ML algorithms (Cantor-Rivera et al. 2015). Multiscale 3D neural network can predict stroke outcome and final lesion contour on day-90 scans using acute stroke neuro-MRI scans taken on day 0. Stacked auto-encoder and deep Boltzmann machine have been proposed for diagnosis of Alzheimer's disease and mild cognitive impairment on MR images (Zaharchuk et al. 2018; Collij et al. 2016).

## 5 ML Applications in Abdominal Imaging

Diagnostic accuracy for appendicitis can be higher with neural networks (NN) and SVM in comparison to Alvarado clinical scoring system (ACSS) (Bryan 2016). The respective accuracies and area under the curve of the ACSS, NN, and SVM were 55%, 93%, 99%, and 0.621, 0.969, 0.997. Characterization of renal stone with ML has been assessed in prior studies, with best reported accuracy of 92% (Park et al. 2013). Data mining techniques such as ANN and genetic algorithm have been applied for predicting renal colic in emergency settings and determining clinical decision rules for patient management. Prediction of spontaneous passage of ureteral

stones in patients with renal colic with ML-based approach had a sensitivity of 85% and a specificity of 87% (Kumar 2012). ML enables automatic and robust segmentation for estimation of hepatic fat on CT (Dal Moro et al. 2006). Recent studies have also reported applications of ML for estimating Pi-RADS scores for prostate cancer on prostate MR (Yan et al. 2015).

## 6 ML Applications in Musculoskeletal Imaging

Musculoskeletal applications of ML have been reported in medical literature. A fully automated ML can segment a region of interest, standardize, and preprocess input radiographs to calculate the bone age from hand radiographs in under 2 s. A combination of traditional machine vision segmentation and CNN technology has been applied to create a compression fracture detecting algorithm for chest CT. Zebra™ (Zebra Medical, Kibbutz Shefayim, Israel) bone density algorithm estimates output from CT images that is equivalent to bone density T-score from DEXA scans (Wang et al. 2017b).

ML has been applied in labeling of rib and vertebrae on single planar CT image to aid interpretation and lesion localization (Figs. 5 and 6). Display of long axes of bilateral ribs in single imaging plane (akin to unfolding of ribs) improved detection and reduced interpretation time for bone metastases from breast cancer on

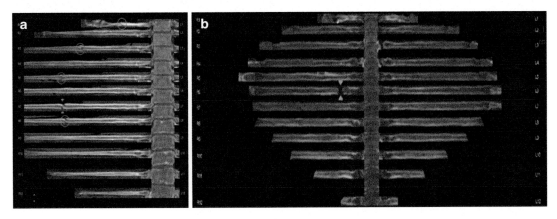

**Fig. 5** SyngoVia™ Siemens software straightens and labels (**a**) the side and number of ribs on chest CT datasets. This can aid detection (**b**) of multiple rib fractures such as the one involving right sixth rib (*arrowheads*)

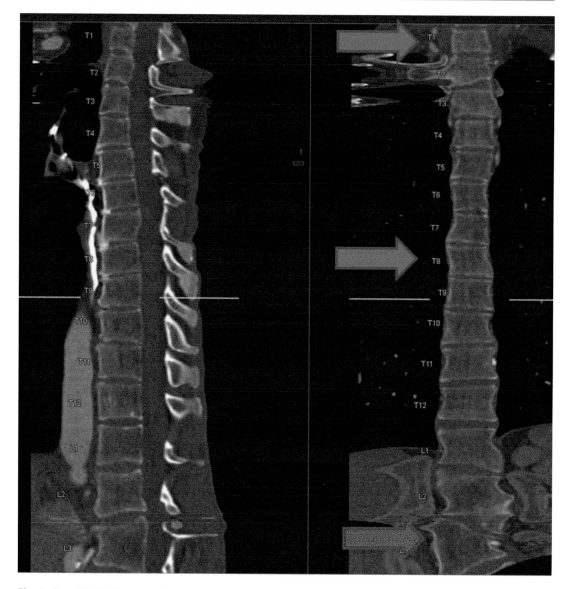

**Fig. 6** SyngoVia™ Siemens software labels and displays vertebrae in a single plane (*numbers*). Anatomic distortion is seen at lower spine (*red arrow*)

chest CT versus radiologists. There was substantial decrease in interpretation time with rib unfolding along with improved sensitivity and specificity for detection of rib fractures compared to CT images without this feature (Ha et al. 2017). Studies have also reported that rib unfolding improves detection of lytic lesions, and aids in evaluation of treatment-induced sclerosis in patients with multiple myeloma (Bier et al. 2015).

## 7    ML Applications in Breast Imaging

ML holds clear-cut advantages in the identification and classification of macro-calcifications in mammography. Studies have reported that ML models can achieve high specificity and AUC values (0.90, 0.90) for analyzing and characterizing macro-calcifications and breast masses. A combination of seven features was found to be better than individual features for differentiating benign and malignant breast lesions on MRI. The seven features included one pathological variable of age, one morphological variable of slope, three texture features of entropy, inverse difference and information correlation, one kinetic feature of signal enhancement ratio (SER), and one DWI feature of apparent diffusion coefficient (ADC). The average sensitivity, specificity, AUC, and accuracy were found to be 0.85, 0.89, 0.90, and 0.93, respectively (Bier et al. 2016).

---

**Key Points**
**Main current applications of ML in neuro/abdominal/MSK and breast imaging**

- Fast cerebral hemorrhage detection and prediction of stroke outcomes.
- Appendicitis and renal colic prediction/ renal stone characterization.
- Hand bone age calculation and rib unfolding for fracture detection.
- Characterization of breast macro-calcifications and masses.

---

## 8 ML Applications in Radiation Dose and Image Quality

Deep learning technologies have been applied to create "super-resolution" images from down-sampled data obtained at ultralow radiation dose (Cai et al. 2014). A deep learning method has been applied for reconstructing ultralow-dose PET data while preserving diagnostic information (Ahn et al. 2018). Siemens Healthineers have recently introduced a ML algorithm which uses a gantry-mounted camera to automatically center the patient and select the scan length for specified CT protocols. Optimal centering in CT helps improve image quality and reduce radiation dose.

Occasionally, suboptimal images are not recognized until many hours after an exam is completed during image interpretation. With advances in ML, there is now potential to instantly recognize, or perhaps even predict, poor image quality, allowing technicians to correct such errors before ending the imaging exam (Rui et al. 2015). ML has also been used to generate higher resolution anatomical outputs (thin images) from thicker 5–7 mm MR images (Itu et al. 2016).

---

## 9 Limitations of ML

Despite encouraging studies, there are concerns and limitations with ML applications in medical imaging. Most ML applications target specific imaging findings or features rather than the entire gamut of findings in imaging datasets. The choice of ML algorithm depends on the data pattern types, hyperparameters, resources, and raw data. There is need for identifying and grouping the data patterns into two or more classes. Limitation of current approaches has been the exposure of the algorithm to mostly the labeled data. Optimal formulation of hyperparameters is necessary to create models with higher accuracy, and data constraints limit the number of hyperparameters (Wernick et al. 2010). The lack of supply of a clean, labeled raw data with verification from skilled radiologists can affect the targeted outcome, thus impairing the application statistics of a devised algorithm. Some of these limitations are being tackled with self-learning and untrained models of ML.

Details of large data-based ML algorithms can be difficult to decipher, which makes it hard to identify errors in image analysis (Suk and Shen 2013; Jiang et al. 2017). AI, particularly the DL, algorithms feed on volumes of data. The digital imaging data will increase to 35 Zettabyte by 2020 as the global volume of imaging studies balloons at an alarming rate of greater than one billion per year. Meeting the expectations of a challenging denominator can be tough, though apparently lucrative.

Most ML algorithms are presently used in controlled situations, which makes their validation in a wider population questionable. The incidence and prevalence of disease, radiological protocols, and equipment are different across the globe. There is also a lack of clarity in the process of FDA licensing, since it is difficult to confine ML in existing laws. Additionally, ML liability concerning clinical images poses challenges for hospitals and commercial vendors, thereby raising concerns about medical malpractice. For AI interpretation to be effective, it needs to meet highest judgement standards especially in critical decisions. Presently, there is lack of clarity in inculcation of complex cognitive factors, thought processes, and reasoning (Jiang et al. 2017).

## 10 Value of AI/ML in Radiology

Despite noticeable advances in AI/ML in radiology with a plethora of validation studies, perspectives, and commercial products, the reimbursement and legal ramifications need strategies and definitions. Studies on how AI/ML solutions will improve patient outcomes are still awaited. Reimbursement policies will likely evolve after such studies and broader more complete evaluation of radiological exams, and then possibly pay for these AI/ML solutions which currently in most cases are not reimbursed. In the absence of clear reimbursement policies, radiology departments face an uphill financial battle to adopt and subscribe to these path-breaking solutions that hold growing promises albeit with an increasing cost since different solutions work on different imaging modalities and exam types.

As a second checker or the first reader, AI/ML does and will help detect, annotate, and quantify findings in radiological exams. This has potential for decreasing medical "miss" rate, improving patient safety (from heretofore missed findings), and quite possibly reducing medicolegal liabilities and insurance costs. On the other hand, legal policies are not clear on AI/ML. These issues have neither played out nor thought about amongst regulatory or judicial bodies at the time of writing this manuscript.

## 11 Summary

Despite lingering challenges, ML has made substantial progress in radiology, from image acquisition and processing to image interpretation applications. With up to 30% rate of errors in radiology reports, coupled with burgeoning use of imaging procedures in modern medicine, and exciting developments in field of AI, it is expected that ML applications in imaging will continue to grow, and one day play a bigger, more meaningful role in improving imaging services, and ultimately the patient care.

**Key Points**

- **Qualitative benefits of ML:** lie in stellar image processing for expediting interpretation, quick interpretation time, time-saving potential for radiologists, and high detection rates (such as lung nodules).
- **Quantitative benefits of ML:** include accurate and seamless quantitation of abnormal findings, and possibly in evaluation of radiomics in oncologic patients.

## References

Ahn CK, Yang Z, Heo C, Jin H, Park B, Kim JH (2018) A deep learning-enabled iterative reconstruction of ultra-low-dose CT: use of synthetic sinogram-based noise simulation technique. Proceedings SPIE 10573, Medical Imaging 2018: Physics of Medical Imaging, 1057335

Armato SG, Gieger ML, Moran CJ, Blackburn JT, Doi K, Macmahan H (1999) Computerized detection of pulmonary nodules on CT scans. Radiographics 19(5):1303–1311

Armato SG, Altman MB, Wilkie J, Sone S, Li F, Roy AS (2003) Automated lung nodule classification following automated nodule detection on CT: a serial approach. Med Phys 30(6):1188–1197

Artificial Intelligence (2017) AI can spot large pneumothoraces on chest x-ray. http://www.auntminnie.com/index.aspx?sec=ser&sub=def&pag=dis&ItemID=119460

Bier G, Schabel C, Othman A, Bongers MN, Schmehl J, Ditt H, Nikolaou K, Bamberg F, Notohamiprodjo M (2015) Enhanced reading time efficiency by use of automatically unfolded CT rib reformations in acute trauma. Eur J Radiol 84(11):2173–2180

Bier G, Mustafa DF, Kloth C, Weisel K, Ditt H, Nikolaou K, Horger M (2016) Improved follow-up and response monitoring of thoracic cage involvement in multiple myeloma using a novel CT postprocessing software: the lessons we learned. Am J Roentgenol 206(1):57–63

Bryan RN (2016) Machine learning applied to Alzheimer disease. Radiology 281(3):665–668

Cai H, Peng Y, Ou C, Chen M, Li L (2014) Diagnosis of breast masses from dynamic contrast-enhanced and diffusion-weighted MR: a machine learning approach. PLoS One 9(1):e87387

Cantor-Rivera D, Khan AR, Goubran M, Mirsattari SM, Peters TM (2015) Detection of temporal lobe epilepsy using support vector machines in multi-parametric quantitative MR imaging. Comput Med Imaging Graph 41:14–28

Chartrand G, Cheng PM, Vorontsov E, Drozdzal M, Turcotte S, Pal CJ, Kadoury S, Tang A (2017) Deep learning: a primer for radiologists. Radiographics 37(7):2113–2131

Collij LE, Heeman F, Kuijer JP, Ossenkoppele R, Benedictus MR, Möller C, Verfaillie SC, Sanz-Arigita EJ, van Berckel BN, van der Flier WM, Scheltens P, Barkhof F, Wink AM (2016) Application of machine learning to arterial spin labeling in mild cognitive impairment and Alzheimer disease. Radiology 281(3):865–875

Dal Moro F, Abate A, Lanckriet GR, Arandjelovic G, Gasparella P, Bassi P, Mancini M, Pagano F (2006) A novel approach for accurate prediction of spontaneous passage of ureteral stones: support vector machines. Kidney Int 69(1):157–160

Erickson BJ, Korfiatis P, Akkus Z, Kline TL (2017) Machine learning for medical imaging. Radiographics 37(2):505–515

Firmino M, Angelo G, Morais H, Dantas MR, Valentim R (2016) Computer-aided detection (CADe) and diagnosis (CADx) system for lung cancer with likelihood of malignancy. Biomed Eng Online 15(1):2–7

Giger ML, Bae KT, MacMahon H (1994) Computerized detection of pulmonary nodules in computed tomography images. Investig Radiol 29:459–465

Gillies RJ, Kinahan PE, Hricak H et al (2016) Radiomics: images are more than pictures, they are data. Radiology 278:563–577

Golkov V, Dosovitskiy A, Sperl JI, Menzel MI, Czisch M, Samann P, Brox T, Cremers D (2016) Q-space deep learning: twelve-fold shorter and model-free diffusion MRI scans. IEEE Trans Med Imaging 35(5):1344–1351

Ha JY, Jeon KN, Bae K, Choi BH (2017) Effect of bone reading CT software on radiologist performance in detecting bone metastases from breast cancer. Br J Radiol 90:20160809

Hammernik K, Klatzer T, Kobler E, Recht MP, Sodickson DK, Pock T, Knoll F (2017) Learning a variational network for reconstruction of accelerated MRI data. arXiv preprint arXiv:1704.00447. https://arxiv.org/abs/1704.00447. Accessed 14 Nov 2017

Hawkins S, Wang H, Liu Y, Garcia A, Stringfield O, Krewer H et al (2016) Predicting malignant nodules from screening CT scans. J Thorac Oncol 11:2120–2128

Hinton GE, Osindero S, Teh Y-W (2006) A fast learning algorithm for deep belief nets. Neural Comput 18(7):1527–1554

Hoog AH, Meme HK, van Deutekom H et al (2011) High sensitivity of chest radiograph reading by clinical officers in a tuberculosis prevalence survey. Int J Tuberc Lung Dis 15(10):1308–1314

Hua K-L, Hsu C-H, Hidayati SC, Cheng W-H, Chen Y-J (2015) Computer-aided classification of lung nodules on computed tomography images via deep learning technique. OncoTargets Ther 8:2015–2022

Hwang S, Kim HE, Jeong J, Kim HJ (2016) A novel approach for tuberculosis screening based on deep convolutional neural networks. In: Tourassi GD, Armato SG (eds) Proceedings of SPIE: medical imaging 2016—title, vol 9785. International Society for Optics and Photonics, Bellingham, WA, p 97852W

Itu L, Rapaka S, Passerini T, Georgescu B, Schwemmer C, Schoebinger M, Flohr T, Sharma P, Comaniciu D (2016) A machine-learning approach for computation of fractional flow reserve from coronary computed tomography. J Appl Physiol 121:42–52

Jaeger S, Karargyris A, Candemir S et al (2014) Automatic tuberculosis screening using chest radiographs. IEEE Trans Med Imaging 33(2):233–245

Jiang F, Jiang Y, Zhi H et al (2017) Artificial intelligence in healthcare: past, present and future. Stroke Vasc Neurol 0:e000101

Kligerman S, Cai L, White CS (2013) The effect of computer-aided detection on radiologist performance in the detection of lung cancers previously missed on a chest radiograph. J Thorac Imaging 28(4):244–252

Kumar K (2012) Artificial neural networks for diagnosis of kidney stones disease. Int J Comput Sci Information Technol 7:20–25

Lakhani P, Sundaram B (2017) Deep learning at chest radiography: automated classification of pulmonary tuberculosis by using convolutional neural networks. Radiology (2):574–582

Lambin P, Rios-Velazquez E, Leijenaar R et al (2012) Radiomics: extracting more information from medical images using advanced feature analysis. Eur J Cancer 48:441–446

Lee SH, Lee SM, Goo JM et al (2014) Usefulness of texture analysis in differentiating transient from persistent part-solid nodules(PSNs): a retrospective study. PLoS One 9:e85167

Lee H, Mansouri M, Tajmir S et al (2017a) A deep-learning system for fully-automated peripherally inserted central catheter (PICC) tip detection. J Digit Imaging. https://doi.org/10.1007/s10278-017-0025-z

Lee J-G, Jun S, Cho Y-W et al (2017b) Deep learning in medical imaging: general overview. Korean J Radiol 18(4):570–584

Lodwick GS, Keats TE, Dorst JP (1963) The coding of roentgen images for computer analysis as applied to lung cancer. Radiology 81(2):185–200

Maduskar P, Muyoyeta M, Ayles H, Hogeweg L, Peters-Bax L, van Ginneken B (2013) Detection of tuberculosis using digital chest radiography: automated reading vs. interpretation by clinical officers. Int J Tuberc Lung Dis 17(12):1613–1620

Maldonado F, Boland JM, Raghunath S et al (2013) Noninvasive characterization of the histopathologic features of pulmonary nodules of the lung adenocarcinoma spectrum using computer-aided nodule assessment and risk yield (CANARY)—a pilot study. J Thorac Oncol 8:452–460

Manikandan T, Bharathi N (2016) Lung cancer detection using fuzzy auto-seed cluster means morphological segmentation and SVM classifier. J Med Syst 40(7):1

Melendez J, Sánchez CI, Philipsen RH et al (2016) An automated tuberculosis screening strategy combining X-ray-based computer-aided detection and clinical information. Sci Rep 6:252–265

Messay T, Hardie RC, Rogers SK (2010) A new computationally efficient CAD system for pulmonary nodule detection in CT imagery. Med Image Anal 14(3):390–406

Pande T, Cohen C, Pai M, Ahmad Khan F (2016) Computer-aided detection of pulmonary tuberculosis on digital chest radiographs: a systematic review. Int J Tuberc Lung Dis 20(9):1226–1230

Park SY, Seo JS, Lee SC, Kim SM (2013) Application of an artificial intelligence method for diagnosing acute appendicitis: the support vector machine. In: Park J, Stojmenovic I, Choi M, Xhafa F (eds) Future information technology. Lecture notes in electrical engineering, vol 276. Springer, Berlin, Heidelberg

Rios Velazquez E, Parmar C, Liu Y, Coroller TP, Cruz G, Stringfield O et al (2017) Somatic mutations drive distinct imaging phenotypes in lung cancer. Cancer Res 77(14):3922–3930

Riverain (2004) Riverain medical introduces artificial intelligence system for CHEST X-RAY early lung cancer detection. PR Newswire. http://search.proquest.com.ezp-prod1.hul.harvard.edu/docview/451600567?accountid=11311

Rothenberg SA, Patel JB, Herscu MH, et al (2016) Evaluation of a machine learning approach to protocol MRI examinations: initial experience predicting use of contrast by neuroradiologists in MRI protocols. Paper presented at Radiology Society of North America, 102nd Scientific Assembly and Annual Meeting, Chicago, IL

Rui X, Cheng L, Long Y, Fu L, Alessio AM, Asma E, Kinahan PE, De Man B (2015) Ultra-low dose CT attenuation correction for PET/CT: analysis of sparse view data acquisition and reconstruction algorithms. Phys Med Biol 60(19):7437–7460

Sohn JH, Trivedi H, Mesterhazy J, Al-adel F, Vu T, Rybkin A, Ohliger M (2017) Development and validation of machine learning based natural language classifiers to automatically assign MRI abdomen/pelvis protocols from free-text clinical indications. Paper presented at Society of Imaging Informatics in Medicine, Annual Meeting, Pittsburgh, PA

Suk H-I, Shen D (2013) Deep learning-based feature representation for AD/MCI classification. In: Mori K, Sakuma I, Sato Y, Barillot C, Navab N (eds) Medical image computing and computer-assisted intervention—MICCAI. Springer, Berlin

Suzuki K, Armato SG III, Li F, Sone S, Doi K (2003) Massive training artificial neural network (mtann) for reduction of false positives in computerized detection of lung nodules in low-dose computed tomography. Med Phys 30(7):1602–1617

Wang C, Elazab A, Wu J, Hu Q (2017a) Lung nodule classification using deep feature fusion in chest radiography. Comput Med Imaging Graph 57:10–18

Wang J, Wu CJ, Bao ML, Zhang J, Wang XN, Zhang YD (2017b) Machine learning-based analysis of MR radiomics can help to improve the diagnostic performance of PI-RADS v2 in clinically relevant prostate cancer. Eur Radiol 27(10):4082–4090

Wernick MN, Yang Y, Brankov JG, Yourganov G, Strother SC (2010) Machine learning in medical imaging. IEEE Signal Process Mag 27(4):25–38

Xu H, Tao X, Sundararajan R (2010) Proceedings of the third international workshop on pulmonary image analysis. CreateSpace Independent Publishing Platform, Beijing. Computer Aided Detection for Pneumoconiosis Screening on Digital Chest Radiographs;9:129–138

Yan Z, Zhang S, Tan C, Qin H, Belaroussi B, Yu HJ, Miller C, Metaxas DN (2015) Atlas-based liver segmentation and hepatic fat-fraction assessment for clinical trials. Comput Med Imaging Graph 41:80–92

Yu P, Xu H, Zhu Y, Yang C, Sun X, Zhao J (2011) An automatic computer-aided detection scheme for pneumoconiosis on digital chest radiographs. J Digit Imaging 24(3):382–393

Zaharchuk G, Gong E, Wintermark M, Rubin D, Langlotz CP (2018) Deep learning in neuroradiology. Am J Neuroradiol 2:5543

Zhu B, Luo W, Li B et al (2014) The development and evaluation of a computerized diagnosis scheme for pneumoconiosis on digital chest radiographs. Biomed Eng Online 13:141

## Further Reading

Artificial Intelligence. https://www.merriam-webster.com/dictionary/artificial intelligence. Accessed 16 Jan 2018

ClearRead CT Vessel Suppress Clear read vessel suppress. https://www.riveraintech.com/clearread-ct/clearread-ct-vessel-suppress/. Accessed 6 Feb 2018

Deep Learning In Wikipedia, the free encyclopedia. https://en.wikipedia.org/w/index.php?title=Deep_learning&oldid=820167804. Accessed 16 Jan 2018 (16:08)

Imaging Analytics https://www.zebra-med.com/algorithms/bone-health/. Accessed 8 May 2018

Turing Test. In Wikipedia, the free encyclopedia. https://en.wikipedia.org/w/index.php?title=Turing_test&oldid=820733440. Accessed 16 Jan 2018 (16:15)

# The Value in 3D Printing

Namkug Kim, Sangwook Lee, Eunseo Gwon,
and Joon Beom Seo

## Contents

N. Kim (✉) · S. Lee · E. Gwon
Department of Convergence Medicine,
University of Ulsan College of Medicine,
Asan Medical Center, Seoul, South Korea
e-mail: namkugkim@gmail.com

J. B. Seo
Department of Radiology,
University of Ulsan College of Medicine,
Asan Medical Center, Seoul, South Korea

**Abstract**

In this chapter, we present six case scenarios uncovering many common questions and issues that we may frequently face in the field of 3D printing in medicine where the radiologists will bring added value through their expertise. 3D printing in medicine is a relatively new emerging field. Therefore, these scenarios could be some examples of applications to find use in everyday medicine. Scenarios including several simulators and surgical guides, which are actually used in a real clinical environment where one can possibly improve the physician's satisfaction and patients' outcomes, are detailed. In addition, the added values for physician's satisfaction and patient outcomes regarding 3D printed simulators and surgical guides are also highlighted. For example, a 3D printed rehearsal simulator of congenital heart anomalies of which surgical correction or treatment, particularly in infant or childhood, is difficult due to small size, its complexity, and individual variation could be very useful for an inexperienced surgeon.

## 1 Introduction

The field of 3D printing in medicine is still emerging with a rapid development of 3D printing hardware, software, materials, etc., which

Med Radiol Diagn Imaging (2019)
https://doi.org/10.1007/174_2019_207, © Springer Nature Switzerland AG
Published Online: 02 July 2019

could be valuable in the episode of care, either through the increase in patients' outcomes or through physicians' satisfaction. Six cases are presented with the purpose to give the reader example cases that could be used in real clinical situations. Radiologists could play a vital role in developing patient-specific simulators and surgical guides for better surgery and patients' outcomes, which needs to start from appropriate imaging. Up-to-date detailed knowledge of 3D printing in medicine is provided.

## 1.1 Partial Nephrectomy Simulator

The 3D printed models are utilized as a simulation model for surgeons for tactile manipulation prior to surgery, or for obtaining informed consent from patients. Producing models with materials of varying color, transparency, consistency, and density has allowed us to overcome some of the problems and simultaneously add reality to the models for more complicated surgery like partial nephrectomy (PN) (Waran et al. 2012).

### 1.1.1 Role of Imaging: A Value-Based Approach

For the aging society, partial nephrectomy becomes more and more popular to conventional total kidney resection. However, partial nephrectomy, which selectively removes cancerous tissue while preserving the kidney parenchyma as much as possible to save functioning parenchyma, is considered a difficult surgery in urology, because a large amount of blood passes through the kidneys that filter out waste products from the blood, and the process of cutting cancer and suturing the remaining kidney's parenchyma without the blood flow should be done in a short time (in general, less than 25 min). Thus, during an operation, the surgeon needs to imagine the anatomical structure of the kidney, such as the position of the tumor, renal artery, and vein and renal pelvis based on the reference image. However, it is difficult to distinguish the precise anatomical

structures using only 2D images such as those obtained from computed tomography (CT).

3D models of renal mass with surrounding normal parenchyma can be reconstructed from a patient's preoperative imaging studies using data derived from multiphase volumetric CT. Especially, accurate and delicate imaging is vital to acquire anatomic information including parenchyma, renal cell carcinoma, renal artery, renal vein, and ureter. For this study, dynamic contrast-enhanced CT imaging after injection of the intravenous contrast agent into the antecubital vein using a power injector at a dose of 2 mL/kg of the patient's body weight and at a rate of 3 mL/s to a maximum of 160 mL was performed with submillimeter slice thickness. The scan delay for the corticomedullary phase scanning was determined by an automatic bolus-triggering technique. Based on these CT images, the renal mass could be reproduced using a 3D stereolithographic printer.

### 1.1.2 Rationale

In renal cell carcinoma management, the objectives of a PN are well established: to remove the tumor with negative margin status, reconstruct the kidney in a manner that will minimize the risk of postoperative complications, and preserve as much of renal function as possible (Hullebusch et al. 2005). For the preservation of renal function after PN, there are two important factors that contribute to the decrease in renal function after PN: (1) the damage of normal parenchyma associated with excision and reconstruction (parenchymal volume loss), and (2) the deficient recovery of the preserved nephrons affected by the ischemic insult (Mir et al. 2013). Previously published reports suggested that the duration of the warm ischemic time was the primary determinant of ultimate renal function after PN, which would have significant implications with deferring to the surgical technique to be used (Becker et al. 2009; Aron et al. 2012; Hung et al. 2013). In most of these studies, when volume loss was added to the multivariate analysis, the warm ischemic interval lost its statistical significance, unless it

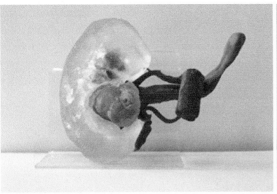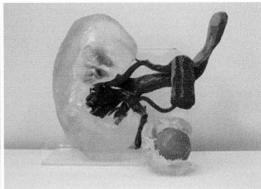

**Fig. 1** 3D printed simulation model of partial nephrectomy for renal cell carcinoma

was prolonged (>25 min), whereas renal parenchymal volume loss has stood out as the most important factor of renal functional decrease after PN (Aron et al. 2012; Simmons et al. 2011; Thompson et al. 2012). Therefore, the ultimate renal function after PN mainly correlated with parenchymal volume preservation, whereas ischemic time played a secondary role. A 3D printed model could be useful to measure and predict both pre- and postoperative renal parenchymal volume (Fig. 1).

> **Key Points**
> - It is difficult to distinguish precise anatomical structures using only 2D images such as those obtained from CT.
> - Especially, partial nephrectomy, which selectively removes cancerous tissue while preserving the kidney parenchyma as much as possible to save functioning parenchyma, is considered a difficult surgery in urology.
> - Accurate and delicate imaging is vital to acquire anatomic information including parenchyma, renal cell carcinoma, renal artery, renal vein, and ureter.
> - A 3D printed model can be useful to measure and predict both pre- and postoperative renal parenchymal volume.

## 1.2 Planning of Aortic Graft

The 3D printed model can be utilized for planning of aortic graft before surgery.

### 1.2.1 Role of Imaging: A Value-Based Approach

Thoracoabdominal aorta surgery is a very difficult kind of thoracic surgery (Coselli et al. 2007, 2016). Basically, the incision range is wide, the accurate measurement of the length of blood vessels needs to be replaced by graft in the open space, and the exact position of the side vessels should be matched. Therefore, the time for the operation is very long and the burden on the patient and surgeon is huge. Even if the surgery is successful, the mortality rate is 6.6% and the complication rate of lung diseases, bleeding, nerve damage, kidney failure, stroke, and cardiac events is as high as 49.8% (Coselli et al. 2007, 2016). In order to reduce the opening time, a patient-specific model for preparing graft with 3D printing was performed.

3D printed model can be used for preoperative planning of patient with thoracoabdominal aortic dissection and/or Marfan syndrome presenting with an aneurysm (Erbel et al. 2014). For accurate and patient-specific anatomical modeling including aortic dissection, aneurysm, and side arteries (such as renal arteries), multi-detector CT (MDCT) angiography with submillimeter slice thickness was used for scanning these patients. Endovascular procedures such as stenting (fenestrated endoprosthesis) could be an alternative with the respective application for this 3D printing.

### 1.2.2 Rationale/Technique

The key points for modeling are to minimize the changes in blood flow to the major organs such as kidney, duodenum, pancreas, liver, spleen, stomach, and spine, which were connected by the renal artery, mesenteric artery, and spinal cord. Therefore, the creation of a new aorta centerline for aorta graft needs to be determined through communication with the radiologist and surgeon in that the blood flow rate in each organ needs to be minimally changed. The modeling is the same as the graft size used for the actual implantation (Fig. 2). The diameter of the aorta graft is 26 mm; each of the renal, mesenteric, celiac, and intercostal arteries is 8 mm; and the iliac artery is 10 mm. After the completed model is printed in the actual size, the sterilization is performed (Fig. 3). As a result, during surgery, a patient-specific octopod graft could be prepared (Fig. 4)

(Park and Kim 2018). Therefore, the operation time was reduced dramatically. In addition, the success rate increased, and no serious complications occurred.

**Key Points**
- In order to reduce the opening time of thoracoabdominal aorta surgery, patient-specific model for preparing graft with 3D printing was performed.
- For accurate and patient-specific anatomical modeling including aortic dissection, aneurysm, and side arteries (such as renal arteries), MDCT angiography with submillimeter slice thickness was used for scanning these patients.
- The creation of a new aorta centerline for aorta graft needs to be determined through communication with the radiologist and surgeon in that the blood flow rate in each organ needs to be minimally changed.

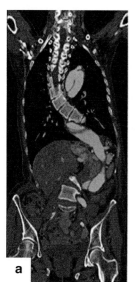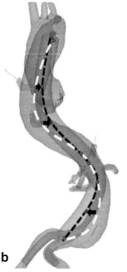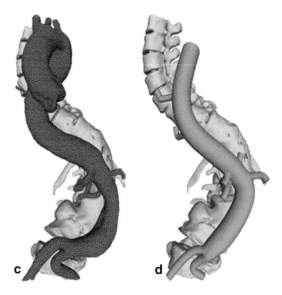

**Fig. 2** The graft modeling procedure for the specific case. (a) CT images and segmentation of the thoracoabdominal aneurysm (TAA) model with severe scoliosis. (b) Comparison between the centerline of a preoperative aorta and that of a postoperative graft. (c) Preoperative TAA model. (d) Postoperative graft model

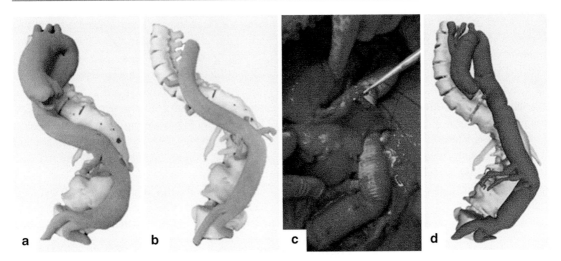

**Fig. 3** A graft guide application for operation of TAA. (**a**) 3D printed TAA aneurysm model. (**b**) 3D printed graft model. (**c**) Open surgical repair (OSR) application of the reconstructed artificial graft. (**d**) After OSR, inserted artificial graft

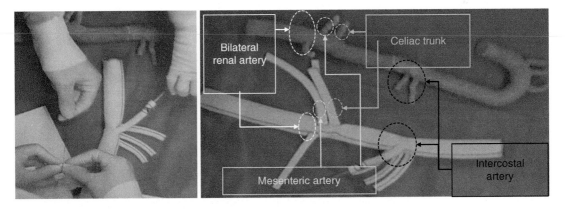

**Fig. 4** Artificial graft reconstruction using 3D printed graft model in the operation room

## 1.3 Video-Assisted Thoracoscopic Surgery (VATS) Simulator

Advancements in technique and instrumentation such as video-assisted thoracoscopic surgery (VATS) in pediatric endoscopic surgery have allowed significantly more complex and delicate procedures to be performed, even in small neonates. However, obtaining a comprehensive view of the operative field is challenging using this technique. Patient- and disease-specific simulator can be made with 3D printing, to overcome this problem.

### 1.3.1 Role of Imaging: A Value-Based Approach

Esophageal atresia (EA) with or without a tracheoesophageal fistula (TEF) is a rare congenital anomaly with different anatomic variations occurring in 1 in 3000 births (Barsness 2013). Over the last 20 years, a broad variety of minimally invasive surgical procedures operated in infants have increased significantly including the repair of EA/TEF. Moreover, in 1995, the mean number of EA/TEF repairs performed by a trainee in North America was 9.2 (range 2–20) (Rowe et al. 1997). By 2006, the mean number of repairs had dropped to 4.4 in the United States (Somme et al. 2012). With few opportunities for trainees to operate any EA/TEF repair, video-assisted thoracoscopic surgery (VATS) for EA/TEF repair may not be effectively taught to advanced level of proficiency within a short training period.

Contrast-enhanced volumetric CT study from 3-year-old patients with EA/TEF was used as the source of the 3D model. Thin-slice image reconstruction (<1 mm) is vital because it has substantial effects on quality of image modeling and subsequent quality of 3D printed simulator. The data should completely include the whole lung tissue, chest wall with esophagus, and trachea.

### 1.3.2   Rationale/Technique

With the advent of 3D printing in medicine, suitable 3D printed models for the purpose of training a surgeon have been created using radiologic data, as well as aid in the planning of complex surgical procedures and in process explanation of such procedures to patients. A 3D printed pediatric patient-specific thoracoscopic simulator was printed to practice a VATS for EA/TEF repair by 3D modeling from lung perfusion CT and multi-material, considering softness and color of each organ for the detailed and realistic simulator.

The 3D models of the lung, esophagus, trachea, and chest wall including bone, muscle, and skin were generated using dedicated software. The segmented 3D images were converted into stereolithography (STL) format composed of triangular surface mesh structure (Fig. 5). The 2 mm wall thickness of the airway and esophagus was modeled by the outside offset function and the fistula invisible on CT was cre-

**Fig. 5** From DICOM images to the 3D model of thoracoscopy simulator. (**a**) Pediatric chest CT images. (**b**) Segmented 2D mask of each organ in chest. (**c**) 3D model visualization with STL format

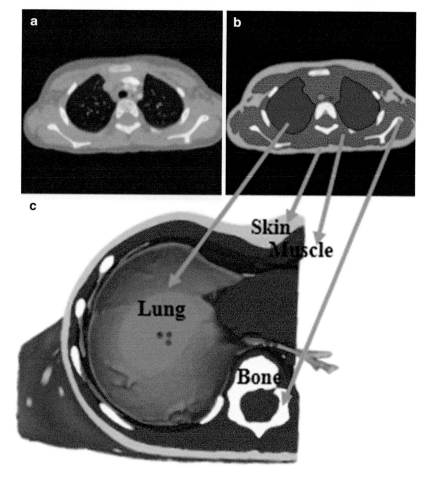

ated using Meshmixer (Autodesk, Inc., Toronto, Canada). Subsequently, artificial seven holes under each rib (3rd to 8th) were created for the placement of VATS ports. The scale of the model was reduced to 80% for matching with that of 9–12-month old infants referred to Korean standard size and the port-hole diameter was set at 12 mm by Magics RP (Materialise, Leuven, Belgium). Using the refined 3D models, a 3D printing model with multi-materials of thoracoscopic surgery simulator was produced using Object 500 Connex3 (Stratasys, CO, USA). This 3D printer offers the ability to print with dual materials to provide a wide range of soft, rubberlike models using Shore A27 hardness, elongation at break, tear resistance and tensile strength, and rigid colored photopolymer material polyjet type with multi-materials of Vero™ color (hard material) and Tango™ Family (soft material) (Fig. 6). The mechanical properties of each organ were evaluated by two surgeons in consensus (Table 1). Simulating of

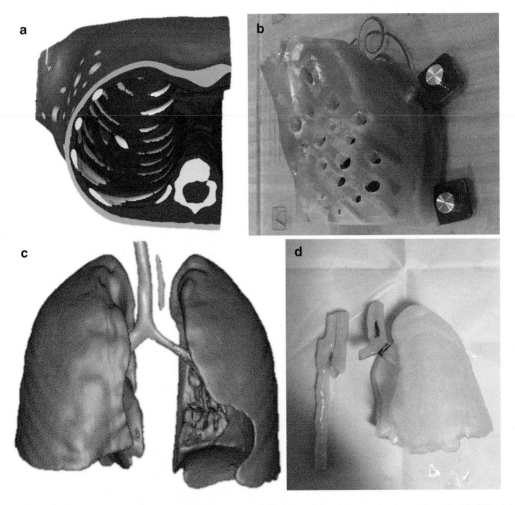

**Fig. 6** 3D modeling and 3D printed thoracoscopy simulator. (**a**) 3D models of skin, muscle, and bone in fixed parts. (**b**) 3D printed fixed parts. (**c**) 3D model of lung, airway, and esophagus as replaceable parts. (**d**) 3D printed replaceable parts. (**d**) can be inserted into (**b**)

VATS using 3D printed phantom by chest surgeons was performed ex vivo (Fig. 7).

**Key Points**
- With too few opportunities for trainees to operate any EA/TEF repair, VATS for EA/TEF repair may not be effectively taught to an advanced level of proficiency within a short training period.
- 3D printed thoracoscopy simulator was able to give more realistic simulation for surgeon training.
- 3D printed thoracoscopy simulator was able to give a surgeon rehearsal surgery in advance for defective area reconstruction with various kinds of operation method.

**Table 1** The various mixture ratios of hard and soft materials on each organ

| Anatomy | Soft material (%) | Hard material (%) |
|---------|-------------------|-------------------|
| Airway | TangoPlus FLX930 80% | VeroCyan 20% |
| Lung | TangoPlus FLX930 100% | |
| Skin | TangoPlus FLX930 90% | VeroMagenta 10% |
| Muscle | TangoPlus FLX930 100% | |
| Bone | TangoPlus FLX930 50% | VeroCyan 50% |
| Esophagus | TangoPlus FLX930 80%+ | VeroMagenta 20% |

## 1.4 Breast-Conserving Surgery Guide

Patient-specific surgical guide for accurate resection of breast cancer can be generated with 3D printing technology based on T1-weighted MR images.

### 1.4.1 Role of Imaging: A Value-Based Approach

The incidence of breast cancer is rising every year. According to a landmark comparative study, there was no significant difference in the survival rate of radical mastectomy and breast-conserving surgery (Veronesi et al. 2002). Therefore, breast-conserving surgery (BCS) has been increasing because the breast cancer has a high survival rate of 5 years after surgery. Especially, BCS has been preferred especially when the size of cancer is relatively small, because small size of cancer makes it difficult to determine incision boundary. So far, to identify the cancer position for operation, a method of clip or h-wire with the help of ultrasonography has been usually provided, but it causes a patient's pain as well as cost.

Among the existing diagnostic techniques, dynamic contrast-enhanced magnetic resonance imaging (MRI) is known as the most accurate technique for evaluating breast cancer (Shin et al. 2011). However, it is difficult to directly use the spatial information of T1

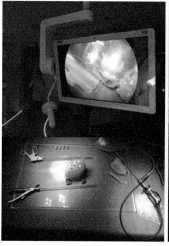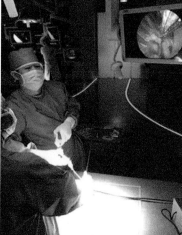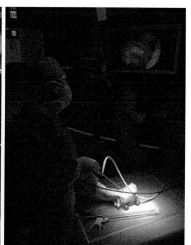

**Fig. 7** Simulating VATS using ex vivo 3D printed phantom by chest surgeons

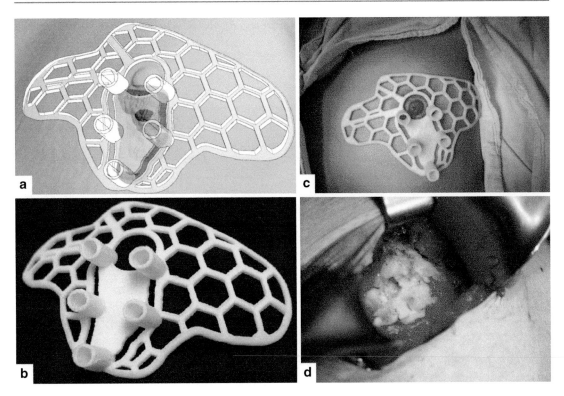

**Fig. 8** Patient-tailored breast cancer surgery guide. (**a**) MRI-based image segmentation and surgical guide modeling results. (**b**) A photograph of a surgical guide printed on a 3D printer. (**c**) Actual patient. (**d**) Photograph of blue dye injection result

contrast-enhanced MRI on the surgery. In addition, inaccurate guidance for cancer margin makes surgeons determine relatively larger surgical resecting region.

Based on the acquired T1 contrast-enhanced MRI, morphological shapes of breasts and tumors were segmented and modeled. Based on breast tissue and tumor models, patient-specific guide for accurate tumor resection can be generated (Fig. 8).

### 1.4.2 Rationale/Technique

The surgical guide was developed to enable skin marking and blue dye injection to guide the location of breast cancer, which allows the identification of incision lines and trajectory in the breast. Based on patient's T1 contrast-enhanced MRI, breast tissue and breast cancer were segmented, their surface models were generated, and a surgical guide mode using these were fabricated by a 3D printer. The method for skin marking and dye injection of the surgical margin including safety area is to design the margin projected onto the surgical guiding surface, fitting to the breast surface. The morphology of breast and nipple became landmarks for this guidance.

> **Key Points**
> - Because of no significant difference in the survival rate between mastectomy and BCS, this last type of surgery has been increasing.
> - This quantitative mapping of MRI information into a patient body promises more exact surgical margins, easier surgery, and shorter operation time.
> - The trajectory of a dye-injection module was designed by adapting a normal vector from the marginal boundary of coronal section onto the nearest skin.

## 1.5 Brain Injection Guide

Patient-specific surgical guide based on MRI images using 3D printing for external ventricular drainage (EVD) can be provided.

### 1.5.1 Role of Imaging: A Value-Based Approach

EVD is one of the most common procedures performed in neurosurgery, placing a catheter for the drainage of CSF to reduce the brain pressure by hydrocephalus or subarachnoid hemorrhage (Mortazavi et al. 2014). In general, freehand techniques using anatomical surface are a common method (Rehman et al. 2013; Abdoh et al. 2012; O'Leary et al. 2000). This results in inaccurate placement, so multipath is used and the risk of infection increases (Abdoh et al. 2012; O'Leary et al. 2000; Toma et al. 2009; Kakarla et al. 2008). MR images for brain segmentation and CT images for identifying accurate landmarks are used at the same time. Skin surfaces and ventricle to be used as anatomical landmarks on T1-weighted MRI can be modeled using mimics and 3-matic© software (Materialise, Leuven,

Belgium). MDCT images with submillimeter were used for skull as a landmark. The skull of CT is registered into MRI.

### 1.5.2 Rationale/Technique

The EVD guide is designed to locate the end of the drain tube at the interventricular foramen (of Monro), regarded as an ideal position, but not to escape the ventricle. To minimize the error caused by the soft tissue of the facial skin, the difference map between the skull and the skin was evaluated and the thinnest positions were considered as fixing landmarks of the guide (Fig. 9). The EVD guide was designed to reach the interventricular foramen when the drain catheter was inserted from the insertion hole of the guide. In order to verify the accuracy of the guide, a guide was applied to the facial skin and the ventricular phantom by 3D printing, and a long bar such as a drain catheter was inserted from the guide insertion hole to the interventricular foramen. The protruding bar above the guide insertion hole was cut and the depth of the inserted catheter measured from the substantially printed phantom (Fig. 10). The EVD guide and

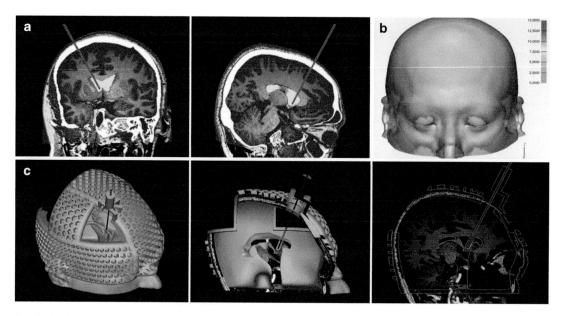

**Fig. 9** (**a**) Segmentation skin and ventricle. (**b**) Difference map between skin and skull. (**c**) A 3D modeling ventriculostomy guide from MRI images

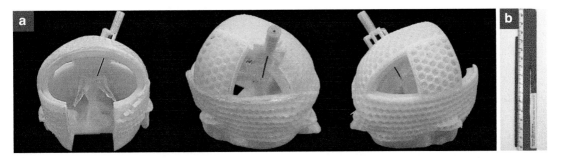

**Fig. 10** (**a**) 3D printer model wearing guide on skin with ventricle. (**b**) 12 cm EVD catheter

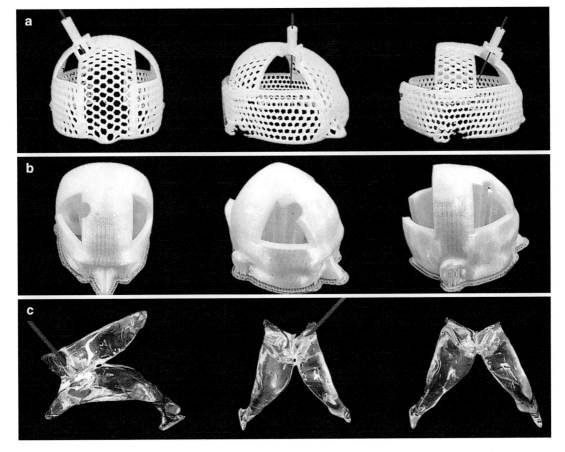

**Fig. 11** 3D printed skin, ventricle, ventriculostomy guide. (**a**) Ventriculostomy guide by Zortrax M300®. (**b**) Skin by Zortrax M200 ®. (**c**) Ventricle by Form 2®

facial skin were printed with an inexpensive fused deposition modeling (FDM) 3D printer with the elastic filament to cover the patient. The ventricle, which was printed with stereolithography apparatus (SLA) printer using transparent resin, was post-treated more transparently to show the interventricular foramen. This intuitively shows that the interventricular foramen is in contact with the ends of the bar (that same length as the catheter guiding length) (Fig. 11).

This guide may help to reduce the misplacement and multipath of EVD in neurosurgeries. In addition, it may be useful for ventriculoperitoneal shunt (VPS) and ventriculoatrial shunt (VAS) in pediatric patients who feel more difficult than EVD in neurosurgery.

> **Key Points**
> - EVD is one of the most common procedures performed in neurosurgery, placing a catheter for the drainage of CSF to reduce the brain pressure by hydrocephalus or subarachnoid hemorrhage.
> - MR images for brain segmentation and CT images for identifying accurate landmarks are used at the same time.
> - The EVD guide is designed to locate the end of the drain tube at the interventricular foramen, regarded as an ideal position.

## 1.6 Congenital Heart Surgery Simulator

Congenital heart anomalies may be diagnosed during fetal heart development in pregnancy, and sometimes diagnosed several years after birth. Surgical correction or treatment of congenital heart disease, particularly in infant or childhood, is difficult due to small size, its complexity, and individual variation. 3D printed models can be useful in this situation.

### 1.6.1 Role of Imaging: A Value-Based Approach

The double-outlet right ventricle (DORV) is a cardiac anomaly where the two great arteries including aorta and pulmonary artery both originate from the right ventricle (RV) and blood from the left ventricle (LV) passes across a ventricular septal defect (VSD) into the RV. In general, occurrence of DORV is less than 1% of total congenital heart disease or about 0.5–1 per 10,000 live births (Misra et al. 2009). Understanding of variation of DORV is critical to choose the appropriate surgical method; nevertheless, it is not easy even by using volumetric CT images.

For newborns and infants born with DORV, CT imaging with a standard protocol is not helpful. Therefore, instructions and adjustment of the scanning protocol by a skilled expert for contrast-enhanced cardiac CT are critical, including imaging time and resolution. The resulting CT images should contain the entire structure of the heart and great vessels, to better identify the vascular and flow changes in the heart.

### 1.6.2 Rationale/Technique

Based on the patient images, a skilled radiologist segmented the congenital heart structure including coronary artery, left ventricle, right ventricle, four valves, and shape and position of the VSD. 3D modeling was carried out with the confirmation of a radiologist. The simulation model was designed for each color representing different regions in order to accurately distinguish the position of the valve and perforation (Yoo et al. 2017). 3D printing materials and coatings of this simulation model were chosen to be similar to the material property of the actual patients for surgeons to perform more realistic surgical simulations (Fig. 12 and Table 2). A 3D printed heart enables better measurement of the diameter and length of the puncture site, which was difficult to accurately measure in a two-dimensional CT image. In addition, the intuitive 3D model could be used for determining the most appropriate surgical procedure considering the relationship between the main operation site and the surrounding tissues. Rehearsal surgery could be performed in advance using this 3D printing model for defective area reconstruction with various kinds of operation method (Fig. 13). In the operation field, the operation time could be reduced, and the accuracy of the operation also

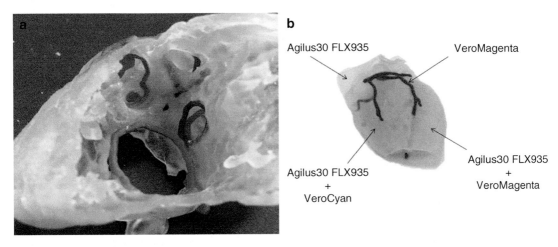

**Fig. 12** (**a**) Valve model with different colors. (**b**) 3D printed heart model with various kinds of materials

**Table 2** Typical composition of 3D printing materials for heart simulation

| No. | Materials | Manufacturer | Composition |
|-----|-----------|--------------|-------------|
| 1 | Agilus30 FLX935 | Stratasys | 70% |
| 2 | VeroCyan | Stratasys | 15% |
| 3 | VeroMagenta | Stratasys | 15% |

could be improved by referring to this 3D printing heart augmented with the main valve and perforation (Fig. 14).

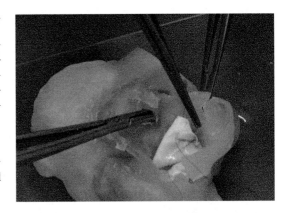

**Fig. 13** Rehearsal operation with 3D printed congenital heart model

**Key Points**
- Instructions and adjustment of the scanning protocol by a skilled expert for contrast-enhanced cardiac CT are critical.
- For realistic simulations, 3D printed model is fabricated to simulate material property of the actual patient with silicone coating.
- A 3D printed heart enables better measurement of the diameter and length of the puncture site, and helps to determine the most appropriate surgical procedure (rehearsal surgery could be performed in advance), so that the real operation time can be reduced and the final accuracy can be improved.

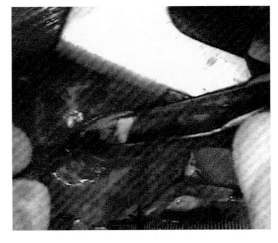

**Fig. 14** 3D printed heart model in the operation room was captured from a surgical endoscopy

## 2 Summary

Radiologists can add value with 3D printing in medicine. With 3D printing, patient-specific simulators, medical devices, and implants from medical images could be fabricated, which could be valuable to various kinds of typical episodes including partial nephrectomy simulator, planning of aortic graft, video-assisted thoracoscopic surgery simulator, breast-conserving surgery guide, brain injection guide, and congenital heart surgery simulator in real medical and surgical situations. Radiologists could play a vital role in developing patient-specific simulators, medical devices, and implants with 3D printing for better surgery and patients' outcomes. Especially, instructions and adjustment of the image scanning protocol for 3D printing by a skilled expert are critical. For accurate patient-specific simulators, medical devices, and implants, 3D printed model should be fabricated to simulate material property of the actual patient with various kinds of materials and post-processing such as coating and sanding. Adequate designed and 3D printed model could be used as patient-specific devices for better planning, operation, and reconstruction to determine the most appropriate surgical procedures, so that the real operation time can be reduced and the final accuracy of surgery and patients' outcomes can be improved.

## References

Abdoh MG et al (2012) Accuracy of external ventricular drainage catheter placement. Acta Neurochir 154(1):153–159. https://doi.org/10.1007/s00701-011-1136-9

Aron M, Gill IS, Campbell SC (2012) A nonischemic approach to partial nephrectomy is optimal. Yes. J Urol 187:387–388

Barsness KA (2013) Collaboration in simulation: the development and initial validation of a novel thoracoscopic neonatal simulator. J Pediatr Surg 48:1232–1238. https://doi.org/10.1016/j.jpedsurg.2013.03.015

Becker F, Van Poppel H, Hakenberg OW et al (2009) Assessing the impact of ischaemia time during partial nephrectomy. Eur Urol 56:625–634

Coselli JS, Bozinovski J, LeMaire SA (2007) Open surgical repair of 2286 thoracoabdominal aortic aneurysms. Ann Thorac Surg 83(2):S862–S864,. ISSN 0003-4975. https://doi.org/10.1016/j.athoracsur.2006.10.088

Coselli JS, LeMaire SA, Preventza O, de la Cruz KI, Cooley DA, Price MD, Stolz AP, Green SY, Arredondo CN, Rosengart TK (2016) Outcomes of 3309 thoracoabdominal aortic aneurysm repairs. J Thorac Cardiovasc Surg 151(5):1323–1338., ISSN 0022-5223. https://doi.org/10.1016/j.jtcvs.2015.12.050

Erbel R, Aboyans V, Boileau C et al (2014) 2014 ESC Guidelines on the diagnosis and treatment of aortic diseases: document covering acute and chronic aortic diseases of the thoracic and abdominal aorta of the adult, The Task Force for the Diagnosis and Treatment of Aortic Diseases of the European Society of Cardiology (ESC). Eur Heart J 35(41):2873–2926. https://doi.org/10.1093/eurheartj/ehu281

Hullebusch ED, Utomo S, Zandvoort MH, Lens PNL (2005) Comparison of three sequential extraction procedures to describe metal fractionation in anaerobic granular sludges. Talanta 65:549–558

Hung AJ, Cai J, Simmons MN, Gill IS (2013) "Trifecta" in partial nephrectomy. J Urol 189:36–42

Kakarla UK et al (2008) Safety and accuracy of bedside external ventricular drain placement. Neurosurgery 63(1 Suppl 1):ONS162–ONS167. https://doi.org/10.1227/01.NEU.0000312390.83127.7F

Mir MC, Campbell RA, Sharma N et al (2013) Parenchymal volume preservation and ischemia during partial nephrectomy: functional and volumetric analysis. Urology 82:263–268

Misra M et al (2009) Prevalence and pattern of congenital heart disease in school children of eastern Uttar Pradesh. Indian Heart J 61:58–60

Mortazavi MM et al (2014) The ventricular system of the brain: a comprehensive review of its history, anatomy, histology, embryology, and surgical considerations. Childs Nerv Syst 30(1):19–35. https://doi.org/10.1007/s00381-013-2321-3

O'Leary ST et al (2000) Efficacy of the Ghajar Guide revisited: a prospective study. J Neurosurg 92(5):801–803. http://thejns.org/doi/abs/10.3171/jns.2000.92.5.0801

Park SJ, Kim JB (2018) An eight-branched aortic graft for reconstruction of visceral and intercostal arteries during extent II thoraco-abdominal aortic surgery. Eur J Cardiothorac Surg 53(6):1282–1283. https://doi.org/10.1093/ejcts/ezx393

Rehman T et al (2013) A radiographic analysis of ventricular trajectories. World Neurosurg 80(1):173–178. https://doi.org/10.1016/j.wneu.2012.12.012

Rowe MI, Courcoulas A, Reblock K (1997) An analysis of the operative experience of north American pediatric surgical training programs and residents. J Pediatr Surg 32:184–191. https://doi.org/10.1016/S0022-3468(97)90176-7

Shin HJ et al (2011) Comparison of mammography, sonography, MRI and clinical examination in patients with locally advanced or inflammatory breast cancer who underwent neoadjuvant chemotherapy. Br J Radiol 84(1003):612–620

Simmons MN, Fergany AF, Campbell SC (2011) Effect of parenchymal volume preservation on kidney function after partial nephrectomy. J Urol 186:405–410

Somme S et al (2012) Alignment of training curriculum and surgical practice: implications for competency, manpower, and practice modeling. Eur J Pediatr Surg 22:74–79. https://www.researchgate.net/profile/Michael_Bronsert/publication/221877752_Alignment_of_Training_Curriculum_and_Surgical_Practice_Implications_for_Competency_Manpower_and_Practice_Modeling/links/00b495242eda802a19000000.pdf

Thompson RH, Lane BR, Lohse CM et al (2012) Renal function after partial nephrectomy: effect of warm ischemia relative to quantity and quality of preserved kidney. Urology 79:356–360

Toma AK et al (2009) External ventricular drain insertion accuracy is three a need for change in practices. Neurosurgery 65(6):1197–1201. https://doi.org/10.1227/01.NEU.0000356973.39913.0B

Veronesi U, Cascinelli N, Mariani L, Greco M, Saccozzi R, Luini A, Aguilar M, Marubini E (2002) Twenty-year follow-up of a randomized study comparing breast-conserving surgery with radical mastectomy for early breast cancer. N Engl J Med 347(16):1227–1232

Waran V, Menon R, Pancharatnam D et al (2012) The creation and verification of cranial models using three-dimensional rapid prototyping technology in field of transnasal sphenoid endoscopy. Am J Rhinol Allergy 26:e132–e136

Yoo S-J et al (2017) Hands-on surgical training of congenital heart surgery using 3-dimensional print models. J Thorac Cardiovasc Surg 153(6):1530–1540

# Incentivizing Radiologists

Florian Hofer, Carlos Francisco Silva,
and Tom Stargardt

## Contents

**Abstract**

There are many different approaches to incentivize radiologists and physicians in general and in particular to adhere to value-based imaging/medicine. These can be divided roughly into nonfinancial and financial incentives. Deciding which approach to take depends in large part on the goals of decision makers. Payment methods are an important way to create financial incentives for health professionals. Different methods—fee-for-service payments, bundled payments, and pay-for-performance schemes, explained throughout this chapter—create different incentives, some of which can lead to unintended or undesired consequences.

F. Hofer · T. Stargardt (✉)
Hamburg Center for Health Economics,
Universität Hamburg, Hamburg, Germany
e-mail: Tom.Stargardt@uni-hamburg.de

C. F. Silva
Department of Diagnostic and Interventional
Radiology, Universitätsklinikum Heidelberg,
Heidelberg, Germany

## 1   Introduction

From an economic perspective, value-based medical imaging requires (a) ensuring that resources are not spent on unnecessary services (i.e., wasted) and, at the same time, (b) maintaining an acceptable balance between resources (i.e., input) and outcomes (i.e., value for money). Outcomes of interest may include efficacy, quality, safety, or patient satisfaction.

As in other areas of value-based medicine, it is crucial to identify a set of financial and nonfinancial incentives to help ensure that resources are distributed efficiently while

Med Radiol Diagn Imaging (2019)
https://doi.org/10.1007/174_2019_211, © Springer Nature Switzerland AG
Published Online: 28 June 2019

simultaneously minimizing the need for extensive monitoring of healthcare providers. Despite the multitude of guidelines and recommendations on this topic, incentives in radiology are still being set primarily within reimbursement catalogs or systems. Until very recently, these have relied, for the most part, on either **fee-for-service** payments or **bundled payments**. In value-based medicine, however, reimbursement is usually expected to depend on preselected outcomes, an approach that is at the heart of **pay-for-performance** models.

The remainder of this chapter will be organized as follows: it will start with a brief review of recent initiatives that aim to avoid wasteful use of resources. This will be followed by an overview of approaches to incentivize physicians on a daily basis using financial lives, including **fee-for-service** payments, **bundled payments**, and **pay-for-performance** schemes.

## 2 Nonfinancial Incentives for Avoiding Wasteful Use of Resources

Over the past several decades, there have been numerous efforts to reduce the waste of resources in the healthcare sector, many of which have taken the form of campaigns. One example is the Choosing Wisely initiative launched in 2012 by the American Board of Internal Medicine (ABIM) Foundation. The initiative aims to inform physicians about evidence-based recommendations, with the ultimate goal of reducing unnecessary tests and procedures while promoting conversations between providers and patients that will help them make informed healthcare choices. To date, recommendations have been released across nearly 20 countries, all of which have a similar amount of healthcare overuse, with roughly 30% of tests and procedures thought to be unnecessary (ABIM Foundation 2018).

A second example, the Image Wisely campaign, was started in 2010 by the American College of Radiology (ACR), Radiological Society of North America (RSNA), American Association of Physicists in Medicine (AAPM), and American Society of Radiologic Technologists (ASRT). It aims to reduce radiation exposure in imaging through a variety of approaches, including initiatives to avoid unnecessary imaging and redundant procedures. Additionally, following concerns about increased exposure to ionizing radiation in the pediatric population, the Society for Pediatric Radiology, ACR, AAPM, and ASRT launched the Image Gently initiative.

In both examples, resources and information are offered to radiologists, medical physicists, other imaging practitioners, and patients to facilitate safe and effective imaging of adult and children worldwide (Image Gently® 2018; Image Wisely® 2018). In the long run, these campaigns and others like them should lead to recommendations that will eventually find their way into common guidelines. With clinical decision support (CDS) software, it may even be possible to help physicians adhere to such guidelines in real time in the near future.

Another important way to create nonfinancial incentives for physicians is to use benchmarking. In the healthcare context, this may take the form of internal benchmarking (e.g., the comparison of different departments within an entity such as a hospital) or competitive benchmarking (e.g., a comparison across different providers). One example of competitive benchmarking is the hospital quality reports in Germany, where hospitals are obliged to provide information publicly on the quantity and quality of services they provide. Competitive benchmarking may be especially effective in healthcare systems where individuals are free to choose their providers, as is the case in Germany. However, empirical evidence suggests that the creation of financial incentives can have a significant impact on the behavior of physicians (Flodgren et al. 2011) and should therefore be used in addition to nonfinancial incentives.

## 3      Creating Incentives Through Different Payment Methods

Although guideline recommendations must always be interpreted and implemented in light of individual patients' needs, guidelines are nevertheless a valuable tool for assessing whether the services delivered by a provider are appropriate. If the guidelines in question take cost-effectiveness and prevention of waste into account, it can be useful to incentivize health professionals to follow their recommendations more closely and thus prevent wasteful resource use ex ante. For this task, some payment methods may be more suitable than others. The following section will describe three of these, namely fee-for-service, bundled payments, and pay-for-performance.

## 3.1      Fee-for-Service

As the name suggests, the idea of **fee-for-service** payments is to reimburse service provision in as detailed a way as possible. For example, if a physician provides multiple services for a patient, each of these is paid for separately. **Fee-for-service** payment systems that have no global cap in expenditures therefore incentivize physicians to increase the overall number of services they provide (although it is possible to set the payments for each service differently and thereby reward the provision of some services more than others). Usually, reimbursement rates in fee-for-service systems are independent of outcomes for quality of care.

While the incentives in such systems are strong, they can be counteracted by financial incentives that are unrelated to reimbursement.

For example, in a recent survey of physicians conducted by the ABIM Foundation, respondents stated that the main reason they continued to order low-value tests and procedures was because of malpractice concerns (Collar and Mainor 2017).

## 3.2      Bundled Payments

Put simply, **bundled payments** are designed to reimburse packages of services provided to treat or diagnose a certain health condition. In contrast to fee-for-service payments, bundled payments do not reimburse physicians for each distinct service they provide, but rather pay a predefined amount to cover the average expense of a clinically defined episode of care (usually consisting of diagnosis and treatment). Depending on the underlying disease, bundled payments can be adjusted for severity.

It is important to note that reimbursement rates in a bundled payment system do not depend on the actual services provided, thus giving physicians leeway to choose which treatment or service they feel is necessary for any given patient. If, for example, an innovative treatment becomes available, a physician is free to carry it out rather than wait until it has found its way into the reimbursement catalog of a fee-for-service system. Moreover, unlike fee-for-service systems, bundled payments do not incentivize physicians to increase the volume of services they provide (Miller 2009). As a result, bundled payments can be used to improve the efficiency of resource allocation. This being said, physicians may perceive bundled payments as an incentive to reduce the intensity of treatment or number of services they provide per patient (Reschovsky et al. 2006) while simultaneously increasing the number of patients they treat. Clearly, this could compromise the quality of care. The diagnosis-related groups (DRGs) currently used in many countries to pay for inpatient care are an important example of bundled payments.

**Example: Incentives Created by Fee-for-Service and Bundled Payments**

In Table 1, we assume that there are two hospitals that are expected to make the same diagnosis of acute pancreatitis. Hospital B follows existing recommendations whereas Hospital A diverges from them. We will now compare the different incentives associated with **fee-for-service** and **bundled payments**.

Let us assume that every service $j$ delivered by either hospital $i$ is associated with costs $C_j$. In the case of **fee-for-services**, every service $j$ that is provided will be reimbursed at reimbursement rate $R_j$. Let us further assume that both hospitals are equally efficient in their service provision and manage to achieve a small profit $P_j$ for each service provided under the fee-for-service scheme. Following these assumptions and assuming as well that the profit is the same for all services across the two hospitals, the profits raised by Hospitals A and B under fee-for-service can be calculated as follows:

$$P_A = (R_1 - C_1) + (R_2 - C_2) + (R_3 - C_3) + (R_4 - C_4)$$

$$P_B = (R_1 - C_1) + (R_4 - C_4)$$

which is equal to

$$P_A = P_1 + P_2 + P_3 + P_4$$

$$P_B = P_1 + P_4$$

Since Hospital B provides fewer services (i.e., services 1 and 4), its profit will be smaller (i.e., $P_A > P_B$). Thus, in a fee-for-service system, Hospital B is incentivized to increase the volume of services it provides so that it can increase its profit.

In a system that uses bundled payments, services are not reimbursed individually. Instead, providers are paid a lump sum that reflects the average expenditure associated with a package of services (in this example, for the diagnosis of acute pancreatitis). Let us assume that most hospitals already follow the existing guidelines. In this case, bundled payments will reflect the average expenditure for services provided in concordance with these guidelines. Therefore, the provision of services will be profitable only if their costs do not exceed the bundled payment $B$. In this case, the profit for Hospitals A and B can be calculated as follows:

$$P_A = B - (C_1 + C_2 + C_3 + C_4)$$

$$P_B = B - (C_1 + C_4)$$

Hospital A still provides more services than Hospital B, but receives the same bundled payment $B$. Most likely, the costs to Hospital A will exceed reimbursement. Because Hospital B provides fewer services, it is expected to earn a small profit. As in any case $P_B > P_A$, Hospital A is incentivized to reduce the number of services it provides.

**Table 1** Services provided by Hospital A and Hospital B

| Hospital A | Hospital B |
|---|---|
| Always requests lipase (service 1) and amylase (service 2) | Follows ASCP recommendation no. 13 in *Choosing Wisely* campaign and tests lipase (service 1) only (Choosing Wisely® 2019) |
| Always requests an abdominal CT scan (service 3) at presentation in the emergency department (ED) "just to be safe or more confident" and checks abdominal pain (service 4) | Makes a diagnosis based on information about typical clinical abdominal pain (service 4) and whether serum lipase activity is at least three times greater than the upper limit of normal (Banks et al. 2013) |

## 3.3    Pay-for-Performance

A newer approach that has been used increasingly over the past several years is the **pay-for-performance** method. Here, reimbursement rates are dependent not only on the services provided, but also (at least in part) on the outcomes achieved. Physicians can either be awarded bonuses or subjected to penalties when acting in accordance with or against the premises of the payment system. While the approach is easy to understand and offers direct financial incentives, it can be difficult to implement. First, it is not always easy to define and monitor relevant outcomes. In the case of radiology, outcomes based on clinical endpoints may not be an optimal choice, as they can only be measured once the whole treatment cycle is complete and also depend on the care delivered by other providers. Instead, it would be more feasible to measure process quality (e.g., adherence to common guidelines) or even, in some cases, patient satisfaction.

## 3.4    Limitations to the Use of Financial Incentives

Depending on their exact design, all three payment methods can incentivize "cherry-picking." If, for example, bundled payments reflect a specific subset of possible procedures for treating a disease, hospitals have the incentive to discriminate among patients, prioritizing those who are in need of fewer procedures. Hospitals could also try to avoid treating "risky" patients, since the cost of their treatment can easily exceed the applicable reimbursement rates (Weeks et al. 2013). In an extreme situation, reimbursement systems based on bundled payments could therefore compromise access to care. In practice, however, the incentives vary depending on the design of the reimbursement system and components of the bundle.

Similar problems may also arise in fee-for-service or pay-for-performance systems. Even in the case of payments made for achieving high process quality, physicians are incentivized to prioritize patients who they anticipate will be most easily diagnosed and treated according to the procedures set out in the reimbursement guidelines, as doing so will allow them to maximize bonuses (or minimize penalties) (Chen et al. 2011). Also, depending on their actual design, pay-for-performance and bundled payments may give an advantage to physicians who are able to standardize processes they expect will lead to favorable outcomes.

As described above, bundled payments create incentives for physicians to provide fewer services, whereas fee-for-service payments usually incentivize the provision of more services. Focusing only on cost reduction (bundled payments) or on increasing the volume of services (fee-for-service), however, is likely to impact the quality of care.

It should also be noted that, for all payment methods, there are almost always incentives to manipulate how the services delivered are documented—for example, so that they are more in line with common guidelines or appear to cover services that have not been (fully) provided. Because of this, any payment system needs to be monitored to a certain extent.

Lastly, payment systems need to be open to innovations in medical treatment and healthcare delivery, as well as offer flexibility to decision makers and health professionals. If it takes too long to (a) incorporate new procedures into existing bundles of services, (b) add new items to a fee-for-service reimbursement catalog, or (c) redefine outcomes in a pay-for-performance system, physicians will be incentivized not to deliver such services. This could slow down medical innovation to the detriment of individual patients and society as a whole.

## 4    Conclusion

In this chapter, we discussed several approaches to creating nonfinancial and financial incentives in the provision of healthcare. Decisions about which approach to use depend on the goals of decision makers, which in turn should reflect the values and preferences of the society. In some cases, nonfinancial incentives might be sufficient to reduce wasteful use of resources. Much stronger incentives can be created, however, through payment methods. Although payment methods will influence the behavior of care providers, it is important to notice that virtually all payment systems also create disincentives. The interplay of positive and negative incentives depends on the reimbursement system and its design.

## References

ABIM Foundation (2018) Beyond high prices: five reasons to continue addressing overuse. http://abim-foundation.org/news/letter-from-the-foundation/beyond-high-prices-five-reasons-continue-addressing-overuse. zitiert 20 Dezember 2018

Banks PA, Bollen TL, Dervenis C, Gooszen HG, Johnson CD, Sarr MG, Tsiotos GG, Vege SS, Acute Pancreatitis Classification Working Group (2013) Classification of acute pancreatitis—2012: revision of the Atlanta classification and definitions by international consensus. Gut 62:102–111

Chen T-T, Chung K-P, Lin I-C, Lai M-S (2011) The unintended consequence of diabetes mellitus pay-for-performance (P4P) program in Taiwan: are patients with more comorbidities or more severe conditions likely to be excluded from the P4P program? Health Serv Res 46:47–60

Choosing Wisely® (2019) Promoting conversations between providers and patients. http://www.choosing-wisely.org/. zitiert 28 Jan 2019

Collar C, Mainor A (2017) Choosing Wisely Campaign: valuable for providers who knew about it, but awareness remained constant, 2014–17. Health Aff (Millwood). 36:2005–2011

Flodgren G, Eccles MP, Shepperd S, Scott A, Parmelli E, Beyer FR (2011) An overview of reviews evaluating the effectiveness of financial incentives in changing healthcare professional behaviours and patient outcomes. Cochrane Database Syst Rev. https://www.cochranelibrary.com/cdsr/doi/10.1002/14651858.CD009255/abstract. zitiert 11 Feb 2019

Image Gently® (2018) Pediatric radiology and imaging. Radiation safety—image gently. https://www.image-gently.org/. zitiert 20 Dez 2018

Image Wisely® (2018) Radiation safety—image wisely. https://www.imagewisely.org/. zitiert 20 Dez 2018

Miller HD (2009) From volume to value: better ways to pay for health care. Health Aff (Millwood) 28:1418–1428

Reschovsky JD, Hadley J, Landon BE (2006) Effects of compensation methods and physician group structure on physicians' perceived incentives to alter services to patients. Health Serv Res 41:1200–1220

Weeks WB, Rauh SS, Wadsworth EB, Weinstein JN (2013) The unintended consequences of bundled payments. Ann Intern Med 158:62

# Part II

# Practical Applications in Specific Areas of Radiology

# Value-Based Radiology
# in Neuro/Head and Neck Imaging

David Rodrigues

## Contents

**Abstract**

In this chapter, four case scenarios are presented where many common questions and issues are frequently dealt in the field of Neuro and Head and Neck Imaging, where radiologists can bring added value through their expertise input, when patient outcome can clearly be improved, like the diagnosis and management of ischemic stroke, thyroid nodules or low back pain, or the help in the diagnosis of minor head trauma.

## 1 Introduction

Four cases, resumed in Table 1, will be detailed in a case-based scenario, taken from our real-world daily practices. The purpose is to give the radiologist or healthcare professional answers or guidance with current evidence-based best medical or radiological knowledge, with the ultimate goal of achieving the most value as possible, either through inappropriate or redundant imaging avoidance, or through a radiological expertise that could clearly improve the patient outcomes.

## 2 Case 1: Low Back Pain

A 46-year-old female, otherwise healthy, presents with a 3-week history of nagging, nonradiating low back pain (LBP). What would be the most appropriate imaging exam for this patient?

D. Rodrigues (✉)
Imaging Department, Vila Franca de Xira Hospital,
Vila Franca de Xira, Portugal
e-mail: davidnuno.rodrigues@gmail.com

Med Radiol Diagn Imaging (2019)
https://doi.org/10.1007/174_2019_212, © Springer Nature Switzerland AG
Published Online: 02 July 2019

**Table 1** Case scenarios to be displayed in this chapter

| Case | Issue | Key points |
|------|-------|------------|
| Case 1 | Imaging for low back pain | Low value in the absence of red flags within the first 6 weeks; early imaging in elderly patients are not associated with better 1-year outcomes |
| Case 2 | Imaging in minor head trauma | Pivotal role of PECARN criteria in reducing the rate of inappropriate CT imaging in pediatric patients |
| Case 3 | Thyroid nodules | Added value of TI-RADS: good performance in identifying high-risk nodules and simultaneously reducing the number of nodules recommended for biopsy |
| Case 4 | Ischemic stroke | Added value of Interventional Radiology in stroke management, namely the cost-effective endovascular thrombectomy which has consistently demonstrated improved outcomes in patients with anterior circulation stoke due to central occlusion |

**Table 2** List of recommendations in Choosing Wisely campaign, regarding low back pain

| | |
|---|---|
| American Association of Neurological Surgeons (AANS) | Don't obtain spine imaging in patients with nonspecific acute LBP and without red flags |
| North American Spine Society (NASS) | Don't recommend advanced imaging (e.g., MRI) of the spine within the first 6 weeks in patients with nonspecific acute LBP in the absence of red flags |
| American College of Physicians (ACP) | Don't obtain imaging studies in patients with nonspecific LBP |
| American Academy of Family Physicians (AAFP) | Don't do imaging for LBP within the first 6 weeks, unless red flags are present |
| American College of Emergency Physicians (ACEP) | Avoid lumbar spine imaging in the ED for adults with nontraumatic back pain unless the patient has severe or progressive neurologic deficits or is suspected of having a serious underlying condition (such as vertebral infection, cauda equina syndrome, or cancer with bony metastasis) |
| American College of Occupational and Environmental Medicine (ACOEM) | Don't initially obtain X-rays for injured workers with acute nonspecific LBP |
| American Society of Anesthesiologists (ASA) | Avoid imaging studies for acute LBP without specific indications |
| American Chiropractic Association (ACA) | Don't obtain spinal imaging for patients with acute LBP during the 6 weeks after onset in the absence of red flags |
| American Academy of Physical Medicine and Rehabilitation (AAPMR) | Don't order an imaging study for back pain without performing a thorough physical examination |

## 2.1 Role of Imaging: A Value-Based Approach

The answer would be, no imaging at all. Nevertheless, LBP remains a frequent reason for emergency department (ED) visits across the world, reaching 4.4% of all presentations (Edwards et al. 2017), commonly ending in the provision of low-value care such as inappropriate use of imaging, liberal use of opioids, and unnecessary admission (Machado et al. 2018). LBP is also the fifth most common reason for all physician visits in ambulatory care setting (Choosing Wisely® 2019). So, not surprisingly, LBP is probably one the most (if not *the most*) repeated topics in Choosing Wisely recommendations

(Choosing Wisely® 2019), reflected by nine associations or colleges (Table 2).

As we can see, a summary or a bottom line of all the above listed recommendations would be not to perform any kind of imaging in the absence of red flags for LBP within the first 6 weeks, which is also in concordance with ACR Appropriateness Criteria® (2019). Regarding the red flags to be taken into consideration when considering foregoing or requesting an imaging study for LBP, one should consider:

– History of cancer, unintentional weight loss, immunosuppression, urinary infection, intravenous drug use, prolonged use of corticosteroids, or back pain not improved with conservative management—which collectively could raise suspicion for spinal cancer or infection

– History of significant trauma, minor fall or heavy lift in a potentially osteoporotic or elderly patient, prolonged use of steroids—could raise suspicion for spinal fracture

– Bowel or bladder dysfunction (acute onset of urinary retention or overflow incontinence, loss of anal sphincter tone or fecal incontinence), saddle anesthesia, or global, severe or progressive neurological deficits in the lower limbs—could raise suspicion for cauda equina syndrome or severe neurologic compromise

In the setting of Occupational and Environmental Medicine, also a frequent scenario for LBP imaging ordering, there is again no reason, either legally or medically, to obtain radiographs as a "baseline" for work-related injuries (Choosing Wisely® 2019).

### 2.1.1 What If Our Patient Was in Their 60s?

It is still common practice nowadays to raise the bar for suspicion in case of older patients, even if "otherwise healthy," when considering imaging for LBP. Age > 50 years is still considered a red flag by NASS in their Choosing Wisely recommendation, although not by the other 8 nor by ACR Appropriateness Criteria. This is in concordance with a recent comparative effectiveness research study (Jarvik et al. 2015a) that showed early imaging was not associated with better 1-year outcomes among patients aged ≥65 years with a new primary care visit for back pain.

### 2.1.2 The Value of Interventional Radiology in LBP Management

Last years have seen a rise in the Interventional Radiology (IR) armamentarium for the treatment of LBP. Traditional nerve blocks have been known for a long time, but radiofrequency (Fig. 1) is nowadays gaining momentum for the treatment of discogenic or radicular LBP, sacroiliac joint pain, facet joint pain, but also for benign or malignant lesions (Raguso et al. 2017; Gilligan et al. 2017; Kelekis and Filippiadis 2017; Anselmetti and Marras 2017; Georgy et al. 2017). Specifically, regarding lumbar spine radiofrequency neurotomy, there is already Level II evidence for long-term effectiveness (Manchikanti et al. 2015).

### 2.2 Rationale

Regarding diagnostic imaging for LBP, a wide amount of evidence found that routine imaging is not beneficial in the case of acute LBP of less than 6 weeks' duration and no red flags

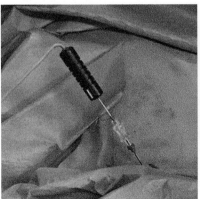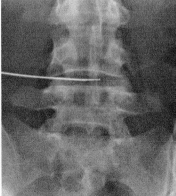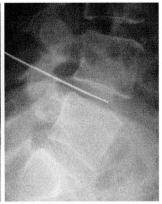

**Fig. 1** Lumbar radiofrequency coblation (i.e., combined ablation and coagulation of the nucleus pulposus). The probe is correctly positioned as assessed by anterior and lateral views [Reprinted by permission from Springer Nature: Marcia S., Mereu A., Spinelli A., Saba L. (2017) *RF for Treatment of Lumbar Disc Herniation*. In: Marcia S., Saba L. (eds) Radiofrequency Treatments on the Spine. Springer, Cham]

(Chou et al. 2009). One should remember that, with or without radiculopathy, the natural history of acute LBP is self-limited in most patients, a significant resorption (>40%) of disc herniation occurs within 8 weeks, and the vast majority of herniations spontaneously resolves within 12 months (Autio et al. 2006).

Until recently, evidence was somewhat lacking for the specific issue of elderly patients with LBP, as they tended to be underrepresented in the literature or trials. But a very important study by Jarvik et al., from the Comparative Effectiveness, Cost and Outcomes Research Center (CECORC) in USA, using a prospective cohort of 5239 patients aged ≥65 years in 3 north-American healthcare systems, found clinically minor or irrelevant improvement in leg pain intensity and EuroQol 5D scores for patients receiving early imaging (Jarvik et al. 2015a). Also, resource use and reimbursement expenditures, overall costs, and spine-specific costs were all higher in patients who had early imaging comparatively to matched controls. Importantly, a higher incidence of missed cancer diagnoses was not seen in the absence of early imaging (Jarvik et al. 2015a).

Regarding the management of LBP, an analysis of the best available evidence—based on criteria including those from the United States Preventive Services Task Force (USPSTF) and Cochrane review criteria—done by Manchikanti et al. has concluded that, for long-term effectiveness, there is already Level II evidence (Level I being the highest, Level V the lowest, opinion or consensus based) for not just lumbar facet joint nerve blocks but also for lumbar spine radiofrequency neurotomy (Manchikanti et al. 2015). A RCT has just recently shown that therapeutic lumbar facet joint nerve blocks in the treatment of chronic LBP shows clinical effectiveness and cost-utility (Manchikanti et al. 2018).

## 2.2.1 The Added Value of Good Imaging Reports in LBP Management

A recent retrospective analysis of 375 patients showed that the inclusion of a simple epidemiologic statement (regarding prevalence of common findings in asymptomatic patients) in lumbar

MRI reports was associated with decreased utilization of high-cost low back pain management (referral to spine specialists and repeat imaging) (Fried et al. 2018). Broadening the scope, a pragmatic cluster randomized trial (LIRE—Lumbar Imaging with Reporting of Epidemiology), currently underway, has already enrolled over 240,000 patients at four large healthcare systems (Jarvik et al. 2015b; NIH Collaboratory 2019a). Spearheaded by Jeffrey Jarvik, this highly acclaimed trial is testing the hypothesis that inserting prevalence data into lumbar spine imaging reports will reduce subsequent tests and treatments (MRI/CT, opioid prescriptions, spinal injections, or surgery). Final results are eagerly awaited, as this study serves as a model for cluster randomized trials that are minimal risk and highly pragmatic. If it proves effective (i.e., reducing unnecessary, inappropriate, and costly care for LBP), it could be easily generalized and applied to other kinds of testing (e.g., other imaging tests, laboratory tests, genetic testing), as well as other conditions where incidental findings may be common. Ultimately, a paradigm shift could ensue, where adding epidemiologic benchmarks to diagnostic test reporting could become standard of care (Jarvik et al. 2015b; NIH Collaboratory 2019b).

---

**Key Points**

- **Appropriate use criteria**: don't request any kind of imaging in the absence of red flags for LBP within the first 6 weeks.
- **Early imaging in elderly patients**: is not associated with better 1-year outcomes.
- **The added value of IR and epidemiologic statement in reports**: clinical effectiveness and cost-utility have already been proved for some IR armamentarium regarding LBP management; decreased utilization of high-cost low back pain management is achieved with the input of epidemiologic statement in reports.

## 3 Case 2: Minor Head Injury

A 3-year-old girl fell from the sofa while playing with her older brother, hitting her head on the floor. No vomiting or loss of consciousness were witnessed, and she did not complain of severe headache. Nevertheless, her mother is very anxious demanding a head CT scan on the ED, as she keeps saying that it was a "serious head striking when she landed."

### 3.1 Role of Imaging: A Value-Based Approach

Minor head injuries occur commonly not only in children or adolescents, but also in adults, ending up frequently in head CT ordering in emergency departments. In fact, nearly 50% of children who visit an ED with a head injury are given a CT scan, but less than 10%, however, show traumatic brain injuries (TBIs) (Choosing Wisely® 2019; Kuppermann et al. 2009). Some clinical decision instruments have been adopted, although with some variability across different practices, with the ultimate goal of reducing the number of unnecessary head CTs in a trauma setting. The *Canadian CT Head Rule* and the *PECARN criteria* are the most widely used, for adults and pediatric patients, respectively, and can easily be accessed elsewhere online (MDCalc 2019).

Specifically for the pediatric population, the PECARN decision instrument is meant to be applied with different criteria for children who are under 2 years old than those who are ≥2 years old but less than 18 (Kuppermann et al. 2009).

No imaging is recommended in children with minor head trauma, with a Glasgow Coma Score ≥ 14 and no witnessed loss of consciousness or vomiting, as in our case scenario. This recommendation is, as expected, in concordance with both Choosing Wisely® (2019) and ACR Appropriateness Criteria® (2019), both based on the pivotal and landmark Pediatric Emergency Care Applied Research Network (PECARN) study.

One should also keep in mind the very sensitive issue of radiation-induced malignancies in pediatric population and try first a clinical observation period prior to the CT decision-making analysis.

### 3.2 Rationale

Released in 2009, the PECARN criteria have since been externally validated in multiple studies, proving to decrease the rate of CT imaging without missing neurosurgical TBIs (Nigrovic et al. 2015; Jennings et al. 2017; Dayan et al. 2017). PECARN is so far the only very large prospective study (with 42.412 patients enrolled) conducted exclusively in patients younger than 18 years old, having demonstrated a 99.95% negative predictive value for clinically important TBI in children ≥2 years old, using the criteria of Glasgow Coma Scale scores of 14–15 after head trauma and simultaneously no loss of consciousness, no vomiting, no severe headache nor signs of basilar skull fracture or severe injury mechanism, defined as:

– Motor vehicle crash with patient ejection, death of another passenger, or rollover
– Pedestrian or bicyclist without helmet struck by a motorized vehicle
– Falls of more than 1.5 m/5 ft
– Head struck by a high-impact object

Of note, the negative predictive value in the cohort of children <2 years old was 100%, and the only 2 children wrongly labelled as negative for TBI in the cohort of ≥2 years old had just a small frontal subdural hematoma (one patient) or occipital lobe contusions (the other patient) ending up in just 2 nights of admission. Clinically important TBI was considered in this study (Kuppermann et al. 2009) to include:

– Death from TBI
– Neurosurgical intervention for TBI
– Intubation of >24 h for TBI
– Hospital admission for ≥2 nights for TBI

Regarding the involvement of patients in the decision process, and considering the anxious mommy in our case scenario, it is worth to note solutions like the R-SCAN project (R-SCAN 2019a). Its aim is to enhance the communication not only between the physicians and radiologists, but also between patients, family, or caregivers. In this project, after consulting the plan with local Patient and Family Advisory Council, clinicians started to educate patients using Choosing Wisely materials and discussed the risks of low-value care. Nursing staff was also involved in this information process, follow-up and help with additional questions. Initially devoted to the problematic of pulmonary embolism, soon it broadened the scope, and now Patient-Friendly educational material regarding *CT for Minor Pediatric Head Injury* is already available for free, online (R-SCAN 2019b).

Finally, but not least, one should also remember that besides the radiation concern, the possible harm of ordering a CT in pediatric population can be the issue of incidentalomas or the sometimes somewhat difficult variant or even normal anatomy in infants, toddlers, or children of young age (Fig. 2). CT reporting by non-subspecialty radiologists can often be tricky, and end in unnecessary downstream tests, surgical consultations, procedures, whatsoever.

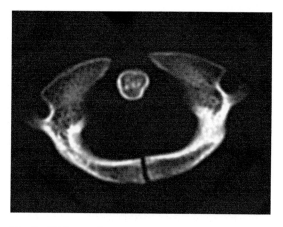

**Fig. 2** CT image from a companion case, depicting an unfused posterior synchondrosis and an absent ossification center in the atlas vertebra of a 6-year-old child. The synchondrosis could be wrongly interpreted as a fracture, in a context of trauma [Reprinted by permission from Springer Nature: Williams H. (2008) *Normal Anatomical Variants and Other Mimics of Skeletal Trauma*. In: Johnson K.J., Bache E. (eds) Imaging in Pediatric Skeletal Trauma. Medical Radiology (Diagnostic Imaging). Springer, Berlin, Heidelberg]

## 4 Case 3: Thyroid Nodules

In a weekly multidisciplinary discussion, the internal medicine physician asks for the radiologist's second opinion about a patient with Hashimoto's thyroiditis who had two thyroid ultrasound reports, performed in an outside facility, showing conflicting data regarding the total number of nodules, nodule echogenicity, size, and management.

### 4.1 Role of Imaging: A Value-Based Approach

The pivotal role of consistency in thyroid ultrasound reports, not just within the institution or affiliated facilities but also among different providers, cannot be overemphasized. Bearing this in mind, ACR recently released the Thyroid Imaging, Reporting and Data System (TI-RADS), the goal being to help in avoid confusion among physicians, ultimately reducing unnecessary biopsies as well as follow-up examinations (Tessler et al. 2017). Dedicated "Macros" or

**Key Points**
- **Appropriate use criteria**: don't request imaging in children ≥2 years old with minor head trauma, with a Glasgow Coma Score ≥14 and no witnessed loss of consciousness, vomiting, or severe headache.
- **Added value of PECARN criteria**: being the most widely used for the pediatric population, they have proved to decrease the rate of CT imaging without missing neurosurgical TBIs.

templates are expected to help in getting standardized reports, but perhaps more importantly, consistency in feature assignment is critical for correctly and accurately categorize the TI-RADS levels (Table 3).

As solid nodules are awarded 2 points for their composition, and hypoechoic nodules also another 2 points, but iso- or hyperechoic nodules just 1 point, it's easy to guess that a vast proportion of everyday thyroid nodules that one faces in head and neck ultrasound practice will be overall within the range of 3 to 4 points, that is TR levels 3 or 4, because frequently found wider than tall shapes, smooth margins, and absence of echogenic foci will not add further points (Fig. 3). That being said, it should be easy to understand that incorrectly labelling an isoechoic solid nodule as hypoechoic could wrongly lead to an unnecessary FNA, even if this nodule measured 2 cm.

An elegant and very educative webinar was just recently released by ACR, freely available online (ACR TI-RADS Webinar II 2019), providing help with practical tips, like the gain and dynamic range adjustments on the ultrasound machine, for better accuracy in labelling a nodule as hypoechoic or isoechoic.

Also, only up to four nodules that warrant further action or follow-up should be described on the final reports, and they all should be measured in the three planes, halo included if present: longest axis on an axial image; largest dimension perpendicular to the previous measurement; maximum craniocaudal dimension on a sagittal image (Tessler et al. 2017, 2018).

## 4.2 Rationale

The issues of interobserver variability, lack of dedicated training or expertise in thyroid ultrasound are well known (Kim et al. 2010; Kim et al. 2012; Rosario 2010). Ultimately, this has led to thyroid ultrasound being handled by some specialties other than Radiology, claiming in small retrospective series a better expertise than the average (Oltmann et al. 2014). We think that for optimal outcomes, not just the number of radiologists performing FNA biopsies should be kept low in a single radiology Department, but

**Table 3** TI-RADS levels (TR 1–TR 5) are based on the added points from the five different categories: (1st) composition, (2nd) echogenicity, (3rd) shape, (4th) margin, and (5th) echogenic foci (Tessler et al. 2017)

| 0 points | TR 1—Benign | No FNA |
|---|---|---|
| 2 points | TR 2—Not Suspicious | No FNA |
| 3 points | TR 3—Mildly Suspicious | FNA if ≥2.5 cm |
| 4–6 points | TR 4—Moderately Suspicious | FNA if ≥1.5 cm |
| ≥7 points | TR 5—Highly Suspicious | FNA if ≥1 cm |

*FNA* fine needle aspiration

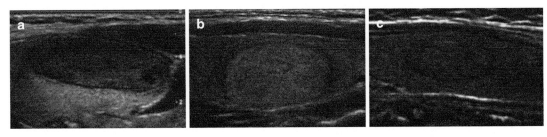

**Fig. 3** A hypoechoic nodule (**a**), a hyperechoic nodule (**b**), and an isoechoic nodule (**c**). Because their shape is wider than tall (0 points), their margins are smooth (0 points), and they possess no echogenic foci, the final score would be 4 points (TR 4—Moderately Suspicious) for the first nodule, and 3 points (TR 3—Mildly Suspicious) for the last two (the hyper- and the isoechoic). Please note that, in case of Hashimoto's thyroiditis, a very frequent presentation, especially in women, the solid component echogenicity of the nodule should still be described relative to the adjacent thyroid tissue (Grant et al. 2015) [Reprinted by permission from Springer Nature: Mandel S.J., Langer J.E. (2018) *Ultrasound of Thyroid Nodules*. In: Duick D., Levine R., Lupo M. (eds) Thyroid and Parathyroid Ultrasound and Ultrasound-Guided FNA. Springer, Cham]

also those who perform diagnostic head and neck ultrasound as well, namely thyroid ultrasound. Dedicated training and expertise should translate into accurate and consistent reports, and ultimately good feedback and acceptance among different specialties who take care of the patient with a thyroid condition. Also, expert handle of ultrasound in general (regarding broad aspects such as physics, artifacts, normal and variant anatomy, etc.) should make it easier to manage challenging cases that sometimes we may face.

Furthermore, the TI-RADS guidelines, although young, have already been tested and compared to others like those from the American Thyroid Association (ATA), and they seem to be gaining good acceptance outside of radiology specialty. In a recent study done by researchers from endocrinology and pathology in Italy (Lauria et al. 2018), it was found that TI-RADS scored high for identifying high-risk nodules. Also in that study, ATA left "unclassified" nodules at relatively high risk for malignancy [ATA was not able to classify a considerable amount of nodules, which showed a significant 7 times higher risk (OR: 7.20; $P < 0.001$) of high-risk cytology than the "very low suspicion" nodules].

Besides significantly improving the accuracy of recommendations for nodule management, TI-RADS has also already proved to be able to decrease the number of nodules recommended for biopsy of up to 41% (Hoang et al. 2018).

---

**Key Points**
- **Added value of TI-RADS**: good performance in identifying high-risk nodules and simultaneously reducing the number of nodules recommended for biopsy.
- **Expertise in Thyroid Ultrasound**: gained through radiological subspecialized training and dedicated teams, is pivotal for achieving the best outcomes, accuracy, and consistency, that ultimately will led to good feedback, respect, and acceptance among different referrers.

---

## 5 Case 4: Suspected Acute Stroke

A 65-year-old man with a history of hypertension and hyperlipidemia presented to a primary stroke center 30 min after sudden onset of weakness on the right side. On examination he had a global aphasia, left gaze preference, right homonymous hemianopsia, right facial droop, dysarthria, and right hemiplegia—National Institutes of Health Stroke Scale (NIHSS) of 22. A non-contrast head CT (NCCT) and a head and neck CTA were requested. A clot in the M1 segment of the left middle cerebral artery (MCA) was found.

### 5.1 Role of Imaging: A Value-Based Approach

In the case of suspected stroke with <6 h, the first steps ought to be rule out intracranial hemorrhage, and to differentiate the extent of infarcted brain tissue (infarct core) and salvageable surrounding brain tissue (ischemic penumbra). The head NCCT is the first line imaging study because of its high speed, availability, and good performance for the first task of ruling out hemorrhage (American College of Radiology Appropriateness Criteria® 2019). The repeatedly validated Alberta Stroke Program Early CT (ASPECT) score can be used to depict the already established infarct core and the ulterior risk of parenchymal hemorrhage following thrombolytic therapy with tissue plasminogen activator (tPA).

#### 5.1.1 Is the Head and Neck CTA Really Necessary?

When possible, head and neck CTA should be done to evaluate for large-vessel occlusion: distal ICA terminus, proximal middle cerebral artery (MCA), the M1 segment, or the basilar artery and identify atherosclerotic carotid artery disease or dissection. This can be done without delaying tPA treatment. The importance of identifying large-vessel occlusion lies in the fact that tPA has low likelihood of recanalizing these vessels, a good target for intra-arterial therapy (IAT). Currently, patients with a distal ICA or proximal MCA clot, NIHSS of >8, and an ASPECT score >7 are often admitted in the angiography suite for intervention (American College of Radiology Appropriateness Criteria® 2019).

MRI offers an alternative pathway for the workup of acute stroke patients. Susceptibility-weighted imaging (SWI) can be as sensitive as head NCCT for the detection of intracerebral hemorrhage (Cheng et al. 2013; Verma et al. 2013), however, is very sensitive to patient movement. The infarct core size depicted on diffusion-weighted imaging (DWI) proved to have a direct correlation with poor outcomes in stroke patients. In general, core infarct volumes greater than 70 mL found on DWI should not lead to IAT given the low likelihood for a good outcome (Lansberg et al. 2012; Yoo et al. 2009).

Nevertheless, one must consider that when a patient is not IAT eligible, MRA/CTA maybe unnecessary or redundant. Doppler US as the initial screening for carotid artery stenosis should strongly be pursued in this scenario. Also, Doppler should be the first step in case of cerebral vasospasm after subarachnoid hemorrhage (American College of Radiology Appropriateness Criteria® 2019).

### 5.1.2 The Added Value of Interventional Radiology in Acute Stroke

Endovascular thrombectomy (EVT) is currently a hot topic in the field of interventional radiology. A handful of recent trials proved better clinical outcomes in ischemic stroke caused by large-vessel occlusion, when using EVT comparatively to best medical therapy alone (Berkhemer et al. 2015; Saver et al. 2015; Campbell et al. 2015; Goyal et al. 2015; Jovin et al. 2015). Importantly, EVT has already proven to be cost-effective (Shireman et al. 2017). Also, a noninvasive vascular study, CTA or MRA, is now a Class I (strong) recommendation in patients for which endovascular treatment is being considered (Powers et al. 2015).

This has led to a joint position statement from main societies—such as Society of Interventional Radiology (SIR), the Cardiovascular and Interventional Radiology Society of Europe (CIRSE), and the Interventional Radiology

Society of Australasia (IRSA)—providing key indications for best practices regarding training or technical issues, facilities, scheduling or availability, expert team and centers composition (Sacks et al. 2019).

**Key Points**
- **Reduce redundancy, reduce costs**: if IAT is not an option, you may consider Doppler US as the initial screening for carotid artery stenosis, which may render MRA/CTA unnecessary.
- **CT perfusion imaging**: useful for assessing if the ischemic territory has sufficient residual blood supply to maintain salvageable brain tissue long enough for successful reperfusion by EVT.
- **Added value of Interventional Radiology in stroke management**: EVT has consistently demonstrated improved outcomes in patients with anterior circulation stroke due to central occlusion. Also, it has already proven to be cost-effective.

## 6 Summary

We hope the reader had a good understanding of these case scenarios, and felt a *déjà-vu* sensation from his personal experience. We hope that the reader can translate the gained input to his everyday life, with the ultimate goal of providing the best and most valuable care to his patient, either through helping the requesting physician choosing the most appropriate imaging for a specific situation, or through radiological expert input in the management of low back pain, stroke, or thyroid nodule FNA.

## References

ACR TI-RADS Webinar II (2019). https://www.youtube.com/watch?v=Y9JU2i4IF-M. Accessed 29 Jan 2019

American College of Radiology Appropriateness Criteria® (2019). https://www.acr.org/Clinical-Resources/ACR-Appropriateness-Criteria. Accessed 29 Jan 2019

Anselmetti GC, Marras M (2017) RF for treatments of benign lesions. In: Marcia S, Saba L (eds) Radiofrequency treatments on the spine. Springer, Cham

Autio RA, Karppinen J, Niinimaki J et al (2006) Determinants of spontaneous resorption of intervertebral disc herniations. Spine (Phila Pa 1976) 31(11):1247–1252

Berkhemer OA, Fransen PS, Beumer D et al, MR CLEAN Investigators (2015) A randomized trial of intraarterial treatment for acute ischemic stroke. N Engl J Med 372:11–20

Campbell BC, Mitchell PJ, Kleinig TJ et al, EXTEND-IA Investigators (2015) Endovascular therapy for ischemic stroke with perfusion-imaging selection. N Engl J Med 372:1009–1018

Cheng AL, Batool S, McCreary CR et al (2013) Susceptibility-weighted imaging is more reliable than T2*-weighted gradient-recalled echo MRI for detecting microbleeds. Stroke 44(10):2782–2786

Choosing Wisely® (2019) The American Board of Internal Medicine Foundation. http://www.choosingwisely.org/wp-content/uploads/2015/01/Choosing-Wisely-Recommendations.pdf. Accessed 29 Jan 2019

Chou R, Fu R, Carrino JA, Deyo RA (2009) Imaging strategies for low-back pain: systematic review and meta-analysis. Lancet 373(9662):463–472

Dayan PS, Ballard DW, Tham E et al, Pediatric Emergency Care Applied Research Network, Clinical Research on Emergency Services and Treatment Network, Partners Healthcare, Traumatic Brain Injury-Knowledge Translation Study Group (2017) Use of traumatic brain injury prediction rules with clinical decision support. Pediatrics 139(4):e20162709

Edwards J, Hayden J, Asbridge M et al (2017) Prevalence of low back pain in emergency settings: a systematic review and meta-analysis. BMC Musculoskelet Disord 18:143. https://doi.org/10.1186/s12891-017-1511-7

Fried JG, Andrew AS, Ring NY, Pastel DA (2018) Changes in primary care health care utilization after inclusion of epidemiologic data in lumbar spine MR imaging reports for uncomplicated low back pain. Radiology 287(2):563–569

Georgy BA, Marini S, Piras E (2017) RF for treatments of malignant lesions. In: Marcia S, Saba L (eds) Radiofrequency treatments on the spine. Springer, Cham

Gilligan C, Malik OS, Hirsch JA (2017) Radiofrequency ablation for sacroiliac joint pain. In: Marcia S, Saba L (eds) Radiofrequency treatments on the spine. Springer, Cham

Goyal M, Demchuk AM, Menon BK et al, ESCAPE Trial Investigators (2015) Randomized assessment of rapid endovascular treatment of ischemic stroke. N Engl J Med 372:1019–1030

Grant EG, Tessler FN, Hoang JK et al (2015) Thyroid ultrasound reporting lexicon: white paper of the ACR Thyroid Imaging, Reporting and Data System (TIRADS) Committee. J Am Coll Radiol 12(12 Pt A):1272–1279

Hoang JK, Middleton WD, Farjat AE et al (2018) Reduction in thyroid nodule biopsies and improved accuracy with American College of Radiology Thyroid Imaging Reporting and Data System. Radiology 287(1):185–193

Jarvik JG, Gold LS, Comstock BA et al (2015a) Association of early imaging for back pain with clinical outcomes in older adults. JAMA 313(11):1143–1153

Jarvik JG, Comstock BA, James KT et al (2015b) Lumbar imaging with reporting of epidemiology (LIRE)—protocol for a pragmatic cluster randomized trial. Contemp Clin Trials 45(Pt B):157–163

Jennings RM, Burtner JJ, Pellicer JF et al (2017) Reducing head CT use for children with head injuries in a community emergency department. Pediatrics 139(4):e20161349

Jovin TG, Chamorro A, Cobo E et al, REVASCAT Trial Investigators (2015) Thrombectomy within 8 hours after symptom onset in ischemic stroke. N Engl J Med 372:2296–2306

Kelekis A, Filippiadis DK (2017) RFN on lumbar facet joint. In: Marcia S, Saba L (eds) Radiofrequency treatments on the spine. Springer, Cham

Kim SH, Park CS, Jung SL et al (2010) Observer variability and the performance between faculties and residents: US criteria for benign and malignant thyroid nodules. Korean J Radiol 11(2):149–155

Kim HG, Kwak JY, Kim EK, Choi SH, Moon HJ (2012) Man to man training: can it help improve the diagnostic performances and interobserver variabilities of thyroid ultrasonography in residents? Eur J Radiol 81(3):e352–e356

Kuppermann N, Holmes JF, Dayan PS et al (2009) Identification of children at very low-risk of clinically-important brain injuries after head trauma: a prospective cohort study. Lancet 374(9696):1160–1170

Lansberg MG, Straka M, Kemp S et al (2012) MRI profile and response to endovascular reperfusion after stroke (DEFUSE 2): a prospective cohort study. Lancet Neurol 11(10):860–867

Lauria A, Maddaloni E, Briganti SI, Beretta Anguissola G, Perrella E, Taffon C et al (2018) Differences between ATA, AACE/ACE/AME and ACR TI-RADS ultrasound classifications performance in identifying cytological high-risk thyroid nodules. Eur J Endocrinol 78:595–603

Machado GC, Richards B, Needs C et al (2018) Implementation of an evidence-based model of care for low back pain in emergency departments: protocol for the Sydney Health Partners Emergency Department (SHaPED) trial. BMJ Open 8(4):e019052. Published 19 Apr 2018. https://doi.org/10.1136/bmjopen-2017-019052

Manchikanti L, Kaye AD, Boswell MV et al (2015) A systematic review and best evidence synthesis of the effectiveness of therapeutic facet joint interventions in managing chronic spinal pain. Pain Physician 18(4):E535–E582

Manchikanti L, Pampati V, Kaye AD, Hirsch JA (2018) Therapeutic lumbar facet joint nerve blocks in the treatment of chronic low back pain: cost utility analysis based on a randomized controlled trial. Korean J Pain 31(1):27–38

MDCalc (2019). https://www.mdcalc.com. Accessed 29 Jan 2019

Nigrovic LE, Stack AM, Mannix RC et al (2015) Quality improvement effort to reduce cranial CTs for children with minor blunt head trauma. Pediatrics 136(1):e227–e233

NIH Collaboratory (2019a). http://rethinkingclinicaltrials.org/news/january-26-2018-the-lumbar-imaging-with-reporting-of-epidemiology-lire-trial-subsequent-cross-sectional-imaging-through-90-days-preliminary-results/. Accessed 29 Jan 2019

NIH Collaboratory (2019b). http://rethinkingclinical-trials.org/demonstration-projects/uh3-project-lumbar-imaging-with-reporting-of-epidemiology-lire/. Accessed 29 Jan 2019

Oltmann SC, Schneider DF, Chen H, Sippel RS (2014) All thyroid ultrasound evaluations are not equal: sonographers specialized in thyroid cancer correctly label clinical N0 disease in well differentiated thyroid cancer. Ann Surg Oncol 22(2):422–428

Powers WJ, Derdeyn CP, Biller J et al (2015) 2015 American Heart Association/American Stroke Association focused update of the 2013 guidelines for the early management of patients with acute ischemic stroke regarding endovascular treatment: a guideline for healthcare professionals from the American Heart Association/American Stroke Association. Stroke 46(10):3020–3035

Raguso M, Marsico S, Fiori R, Masala S (2017) Discogenic low back pain and radicular pain: therapeutic strategies and role of radio-frequency techniques. In: Marcia S, Saba L (eds) Radiofrequency treatments on the spine. Springer, Cham

Rosario PW (2010) Ultrasonography for the follow-up of patients with papillary thyroid carcinoma: how important is the operator? Thyroid 20(7):833–834

R-SCAN (2019a). http://www.choosingwisely.org/resources/updates-from-the-field/r-scan-project-designed-with-patients/. Accessed 2 Feb 2019

R-SCAN (2019b). https://rscan.org/resources-landing/topic-specific-resources/ct-for-minor-pediatric-head-injury. Accessed 2 Feb 2019

Sacks D, van Overhagen H, van Zwam WH et al (2019) The role of interventional radiologists in acute ischemic stroke interventions: a joint position statement from the Society of Interventional Radiology, the Cardiovascular and Interventional Radiology Society of Europe, and the Interventional Radiology Society of Australasia. J Vasc Interv Radiol 30(2):131–133

Saver JL, Goyal M, Bonafe A et al, SWIFT PRIME Investigators (2015) Stentretriever thrombectomy after intravenous t-PA vs. t-PA alone in stroke. N Engl J Med 372:2285–2295

Shireman TI, Wang K, Saver JL et al, SWIFT PRIME Investigators (2017) Cost-effectiveness of Solitaire stent retriever thrombectomy for acute ischemic stroke: results from the SWIFT-PRIME Trial (Solitaire With the Intention for Thrombectomy as Primary Endovascular Treatment for Acute Ischemic Stroke). Stroke 48:379–387

Tessler FN, Middleton WD, Grant EG et al (2017) ACR thyroid imaging, reporting and data system (TI-RADS): white paper of the ACR TI-RADS committee. J Am Coll Radiol 14(5):587–595

Tessler FN, Middleton WD, Grant EG (2018) Thyroid imaging reporting and data system (TI-RADS): a user's guide. Radiology 287(1):29–36

Verma RK, Kottke R, Andereggen L et al (2013) Detecting subarachnoid hemorrhage: comparison of combined FLAIR/SWI versus CT. Eur J Radiol 82(9):1539–1545

Yoo AJ, Verduzco LA, Schaefer PW, Hirsch JA, Rabinov JD, Gonzalez RG (2009) MRI-based selection for intra-arterial stroke therapy: value of pretreatment diffusion-weighted imaging lesion volume in selecting patients with acute stroke who will benefit from early recanalization. Stroke 40(6):2046–2054

# Value-Based Radiology
# in Thoracic Imaging

Carlos Francisco Silva and Hans-Ulrich Kauczor

## Contents

C. F. Silva (✉) · H.-U. Kauczor
Department of Diagnostic and Interventional
Radiology, Translational Lung Research Center
(TLRC), German Lung Research Center (DZL),
University Hospital Heidelberg, Heidelberg, Germany
e-mail: Carlos.dasilva@med.uni-heidelberg.de

**Abstract**

Based on seven case scenarios encompassing nearly 20 common clinical questions in chest radiology the added value achieved through expertise input is demonstrated. The scenarios address situations where thoracic MRI can clearly improve patient outcomes through avoidance of surgical thymectomy once a non-surgical lesion is depicted, or the added value in reducing avoidable radiation exposure and improving patient safety and healthcare quality when choosing the best protocol for cancer staging and follow-up with chest CT. Also, scenarios where the radiologist can add value, mainly through helping to reduce redundancy or unnecessary imaging, that is, in the end reducing the final healthcare costs, such as the reduction of daily chest imaging in the ICU and tailored chest imaging in the preoperative setting or in blunt thoracic trauma without risk factors, are exemplified.

## 1   Introduction

Thoracic imaging is an ever-evolving field, very rich and dense in the continuous update of key useful information, that one should try to translate to everyday practice in order to achieve the best value in the episode of care, either through better outcomes (the equation numerator) or through cost reduction (the equation

Med Radiol Diagn Imaging (2019)
https://doi.org/10.1007/174_2018_206, © Springer Nature Switzerland AG
Published Online: 02 July 2019

**Table 1** Case scenarios displayed in this chapter

| Case | Issue | Key points |
|---|---|---|
| Case 1 | Chest X-ray in daily routine ICU workup | No evidence to support such habit |
| Case 2 | Chest X-ray in preoperative workup | No evidence to support the indiscriminate ordering |
| Case 3 | Chest X-ray in ARDS | Most of the times sufficient for the initial diagnosis |
| Case 4 | Chest X-ray in tuberculosis | Most of the times sufficient for the initial workup |
| Case 5 | Acute respiratory illness | Key initial use of chest X-ray |
| Case 6 | Blunt trauma and mediastinal mass | NEXUS Chest CT decision instrument; added value of MRI for mediastinal masses |
| Case 7 | Cancer staging and follow-up protocols | Single acquisition protocols are best; avoid fasting |

denominator). Seven cases, resumed in Table 1, will be demonstrated with the purpose to give the radiologist or healthcare professional a clear vision of scenarios that one can frequently face in everyday routine work. In other words, case scenarios that have led us to question ourselves if that was really the best option, the best or most appropriate imaging test. Answers and guidance with current evidence-based best medical or radiological knowledge will be provided.

## 2     Case 1: Chest X-Ray in Daily Routine ICU Workup

A 32-year-old female was submitted to an elective laparoscopic cholecystectomy. Besides cholelithiasis and overweight she was otherwise healthy. The surgery was eventful. She developed abdominal sepsis with abscess, further complicated with ARDS and ICU admission. Daily chest X-rays are being requested, from the ICU, stating "routine" in the electronic order form.

### 2.1     Role of Imaging: A Value-Based Approach

Daily routine chest X-ray (CXR) performed in the ICU is still a common standard practice in many institutions, often deriving from solidly entrenched habit or local expert opinion claiming the importance of unsuspected findings in the stable patient. However, strong evidence derived from many studies in the last decade has shown

the low value of such measure, leading ACR Appropriateness Criteria (in last 2014 revision) to state when are chest radiographs appropriate in the ICU setting (American College of Radiology Appropriateness Criteria® 2018):

– In case the ICU patient has a clinical condition worsening
– In case of device post-insertion management (tubes, catheters, or any other life support item)
– Admission or transfer to ICU

In addition, unless indicated by clinical presentation, a routine CXR is not recommended following the removal of a chest tube (American College of Radiology Appropriateness Criteria® 2018).

### 2.2     Rationale

A meta-analysis of eight clinical trials (two randomized and six observational) was published in 2010 by Oba and Zaza (2010), comprising 7078 ICU patients, half of whom received daily CXR and the other half of whom received only on-demand CXR. They found that elimination of routine daily CXR did not increase adverse outcomes in ICU's adult patients, like mortality, length of stay in the hospital or ICU, or ventilator days. Not comprised in this meta-analysis was an important French large multicenter (18 hospitals, 21 ICUs) prospective trial with a cluster-randomized, open-label crossover design, published in 2009 by Hejblum et al. (2009). They found a statistically significant 32% reduction in CXR use in the on-demand arm, without sacrificing safety or quality of care. In 2012, Lakhal et al. (2012), broadening the scope now involving 104 French ICUs, published their prospective observational study, where once again it was found that the on-demand strategy was of higher clinical value.

More recently, in an elegant work by Keveson et al. (2017), from the University of Vermont Medical Center, it was demonstrated how a program of education to the ICU staff about the low diagnostic yield of automated daily CXRs has translated into a significant reduction in CXR ordering. Importantly, there was no increase in reported adverse events, and they estimated annual savings of $191 600 to $224 200.

> **Key Points**
> • **Increase value, reduce radiation, reduce costs**: Hundreds of thousands of dollars could be saved annually by a single hospital without any compromise to patient safety, ICU mortality, or length of stay if one abolishes the culture of daily chest imaging in the ICU.

## 3      Case 2: Chest X-Ray in Preoperative Workup

The same 32-year-old female from the previous case scenario (submitted to an elective laparoscopic cholecystectomy) was found to have a CXR done preoperatively, available on the local institutional PACS, while the attending radiologist was reporting the CXR ordered by the ICU.

## 3.1      Role of Imaging: A Value-Based Approach

Regarding the issue of preoperative "routine" CXR, numerous studies have also demonstrated lack of supportive evidence for their wide ordering

(American College of Radiology Appropriateness Criteria® 2018). According to ACR (American College of Radiology Appropriateness Criteria® 2018; Choosing Wisely® 2018), it is reasonable to order only if:

- There is a history of chronic stable cardiopulmonary disease in a patient >70 years old who hasn't done a chest radiograph in the last 6 months.
- The patient and the procedure present a context of special risk factors, e.g., acute or potentially unstable chronic cardiopulmonary disease, unreliable history and physical examination, and high-risk surgery.

These recommendations are in concordance with the current practice advisory from the American Society of Anesthesiologists (ASA) that clearly states that in cases of extremes of age, smoking, recent upper respiratory tract infection, cardiac disease, or chronic obstructive pulmonary disease (COPD), preoperative chest radiograph is not necessarily indicated (Committee on Standards and Practice Parameters 2012). The Institute for Clinical Systems Improvement, an independent, nonprofit healthcare improvement organization, based on Minnesota (USA), with multiple partnerships in evidence-based medicine among their stakeholder's network (e.g., Mayo Clinic), also states in their local practice guideline that preoperative chest radiograph may only be considered for patients with signs or symptoms suggesting new or unstable cardiopulmonary disease (Danielson et al. 2012).

## 3.2      Rationale

The decision to choose 70 years as the threshold by ACR was mainly based on the landmark systematic review by Joo et al. (2005), published in 2005, who concluded that:

- As the prevalence of CXR abnormalities is low in patients <70 years old, it shouldn't be performed for patients in this age group without risk factors.

- For patients >70 years old, there was insufficient evidence for or against performance of routine CXRs.

So, the prudent and conservative decision by ACR to recommend CXR for patients >70 years old who have chronic stable cardiopulmonary disease and haven't done a chest radiograph in the last 6 months was derived.

Nevertheless, it is well stated that the ability of a preoperative CXR to predict postoperative complications is low (American College of Radiology Appropriateness Criteria® 2018) and that an association between preoperative screening CXRs and decrease in morbidity or mortality cannot be established (Joo et al. 2005). Still, there is currently a tendency to lower the bar and to order preoperative CXR for the patients in their 50s or 60s because of known cardiac disease, although being in the vast majority of times stable.

Considering the scenario of a high-risk surgery (e.g., cardiac), ACR once again in a prudent and conservative approach states that it is reasonable to order a preoperative CXR. This rationale could derive from the lack of evidence regarding the specific topic of cardiac surgery, because the main data comes from studies comprising the more frequent low- and intermediate-risk noncardiac surgery.

Interestingly, only recently a pioneer Dutch study (den Harder et al. 2018) for the first time investigated the frequency and types of abnormalities on routinely performed preoperative CXR in patients scheduled to undergo cardiac surgery, alongside with the effect of the preoperative CXR on planned surgery. This retrospective cohort study included 1136 patients, and it was shown that the majority of patients had at least one abnormality (cardiomegaly, aortic elongation, calcifications, etc.), but in only two

of them (0.2%) the CXR led to surgery postponement, whereas in none of the patients the surgery was cancelled (den Harder et al. 2018). In those two patients with surgery postponement, a pneumonia and a pleural effusion, respectively, could have been suspected based on the clinical and laboratorial findings, or in other words an acute respiratory illness was already present that would prompt both a CXR ordering and a surgery postponement. Also, in this particular case the CXR could even have been requested under the algorithms of *Acute Respiratory Illness* or *Dyspnea of Cardiac Origin* in most common clinical decision support (CDS) tools, and not necessarily in *Preoperative CXR*.

> **Key Points**
> - **Preoperative CXR could be regarded as appropriate when**:
>   - An outpatient presents concomitantly with an acute or unstable cardiorespiratory illness (pneumonia, pleural effusion, acute decompensated heart failure, etc.)
>   - The history and/or physical examination are unreliable (noncooperative patient, etc.)
> - **Extremes of age, e.g., >70 years old, alone** should not be seen as a sufficient reason for ordering a preoperative CXR.
> - **Preoperative CXR for high-risk cardiac surgery**: maybe hard to justify for the stable outpatient; the acute or unstable inpatient is expected to have already had an admission CXR or a full cardiothoracic imaging workup recently before the surgery that should preclude another redundant preoperative CXR.

# 4 Case 3: Chest X-Ray in ARDS

A 52-year-old male presented to the ED with an acute typical epigastric pain, radiating to the back, and a lipase level >3× the upper limit. He had a prior history of high alcohol consumption, but no current or past evidence of cardiac or lung disease. He was admitted with a diagnosis of acute pancreatitis. His condition progressively worsened during the first 4 days after admission with multi-organ failure and acute respiratory illness, prompting the first abdominal CT scan and the first CXR, both ordered by the middle of his first week of in-hospital stay. Necrotizing pancreatitis and bilateral pulmonary opacities were depicted by imaging.

## 4.1 Role of Imaging: A Value-Based Approach

No routine chest radiograph was ordered for this patient on admission. This can be considered appropriate as there were only abdominal symptoms and no current or past evidence of cardiac or lung disease at ED presentation, and is in keeping with best practices regarding ordering of CXR (American College of Radiology Appropriateness Criteria® 2018; Choosing Wisely® 2018). In the same context, the abdominal CT was correctly ordered by the middle of the first week (Banks et al. 2013; Thoeni 2015). If a typical abdominal pain and a lipase (or amylase) level three times greater than the upper limit of normal are present, there is no need for CT for the initial diagnosis of acute pancreatitis (Banks et al. 2013). The ideal time for scanning complications with CT is after 72 h from onset of symptoms (Thoeni 2015). In this regard, one should remember the big percentage (35–50%) of hospital deaths occurring within the first week after admission in severe pancreatitis, in most cases related to lung damage. Indeed, ARDS represents the most common

and earliest organ dysfunction in this setting (Zhou et al. 2010).

- **Risk factors for ARDS—indirect lung injury**: Sepsis; polytrauma; acute pancreatitis; transfusion reactions; drug overdose; burns.
- **Risk factors for ARDS—direct lung injury**: Pneumonia; aspiration or inhalation injury; lung contusion; fat, air, or amniotic emboli; exacerbation of UIP; reperfusion or reexpansion edema.
- **The Four Pillars of the 2012 Berlin Definition of ARDS** (Ranieri et al. 2012):
  - **Timing**: Respiratory symptoms must be present within 1 week after a known clinical insult.
  - **Chest imaging**: Bilateral opacities on CXR *or* CT scan—not fully explained by effusions, atelectasis, or nodules.
  - **Origin of edema**: Respiratory failure must not be fully explained by neither heart failure nor fluid overload; *if no risk factor is present*: then an objective assessment (e.g., echocardiography) is needed to exclude hydrostatic edema.
  - **Oxygenation**: Severity stratified (mild, moderate, and severe) according to the $PaO_2/FiO_2$ ratio, with a PEEP $\geq 5$ cm $H_2O$ (or CPAP $\geq 5$ cm $H_2O$ in case of mild ARDS).

The emergent CXR, ordered next day after the abdominal CT, given a progressively superimposed acute respiratory illness in this patient, was reported with the main findings of "diffuse bilateral lung opacities, no enlarged

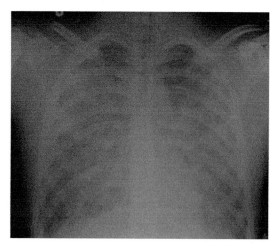

**Fig. 1** CXR depicting bilateral opacities not fully explained by effusions, atelectasis, or nodules is sufficient for the initial diagnosis of ARDS. This CXR is from a companion case [reprinted by permission from Springer Nature: Bassi G.L., Sanussi T., Pelosi P., Ranzani O.T. (2017) Pulmonary Infections in Acute Respiratory Distress Syndrome. In: Chiumello D. (eds) Acute Respiratory Distress Syndrome. Springer, Cham. DOI: https://doi.org/10.1007/978-3-319-41852-0_20]

cardiac silhouette, no pleural effusion, no signs of vascular congestion, no pneumothorax, no atelectasis" (Fig. 1) clearly indicative of ARDS.

## 4.2 Rationale

The current Berlin definition of ARDS, published in 2012 by the ARDS Definition Task Force, clearly states that bilateral opacities not fully explained by effusions, atelectasis, or nodules can be evidenced by CXR alone (Ranieri et al. 2012). So, with the clear-cut CXR findings encountered in our clinical scenario together with the clinical and ventilation parameters, there is a clear diagnosis of ARDS. An additional confirmation using CT demonstrating widespread diffuse alveolar damage is not required. More recently, in 2017, American Thoracic Society (ATS), European Society of Intensive Care Medicine (ESICM), and Society of Critical Care Medicine (SCCM) joined efforts to publish a guideline about mechanical

ventilation on ARDS (Fan et al. 2017). The main recommendations were:

- To favor the use of lower tidal volumes and lower inspiratory pressures, and also the use of prone positioning (for more than 12 h/day) in severe ARDS.
- To avoid routine use of high-frequency oscillatory ventilation in moderate/severe ARDS.
- High PEEP or recruitment maneuvers in moderate/severe ARDS (conditional recommendations).
- About ECMO in severe ARDS (no current evidence to support or avoid it).

Spearheaded by Eddy Fan, this entire manuscript (Fan et al. 2017) does not make a single mention to computed tomography regarding the abovementioned topics of tidal volumes, recruitment maneuvers, PEEP management, whatsoever. After this, even more recently, the same author as well as Bernard GR (the spearhead in the first ARDS definition published in 1994) currently continue to address uncertainties regarding the added value of CT imaging in the initial diagnosis of ARDS and in the ventilator management guidance (Fan et al. 2018; Ware et al. 2017). The doubts about the true pathological and/or treatment mechanisms in the bilateral opacities depicted by CXR lead to the consideration of completely removing the *Chest Imaging* criteria in ARDS definition in future revisions, or its replacement by ultrasound or chest CT, once they prove more reliable in future trials (Fan et al. 2018).

Let's be clear: if everything is obvious and ventilation is running as expected without any discrepancies or difficulties, CT is not required. If something is inconclusive or not explained by vital parameters or lab results, CT is logically appropriate. So, in the less frequent, non-straightforward case scenarios, without an obvious cause for ARDS, chest CT has its role. It can point towards a pulmonary cause if presenting opacities are asymmetric, or towards an extrapulmonary cause if symmetric (Goodman et al. 1999).

Blood analytics including common markers of immunologic diseases, bronchoalveolar lavage or even biopsy might be further diagnostic options, if ARDS persists without any infectious proof or other apparent etiology. In this regard, CT-oriented biopsy could also be helpful increasing the yield of histopathological interpretation. Also, in the longitudinal follow-up of ARDS patients, CT can be valuable demonstrating possible sequela from ventilation (barotrauma) or from the disease itself (fibrotic changes, bronchiectasis, etc.).

---

**Key Points**

- **Appropriateness of request**: A chest X-ray depicting bilateral opacities not fully explained by effusions, atelectasis, or nodules is sufficient for the initial diagnosis of ARDS in the straightforward clinical setting.
- **ARDS underrecognition**: Missing rates as high as 52–69% are still currently reported in clinical grounds when all the criteria for ARDS are already present (Ferguson et al. 2005; Fröhlich et al. 2013). The radiologist is often the first to point to this diagnosis.
- **Admission or transfer to ICU**: Only a chest X-ray is to be considered or recommended rated 7 on the 9-point scale of the ACR Appropriateness Criteria (2018), if not yet done for the patient with acute respiratory illness.

---

## 5 Case 4: Chest X-Ray in Tuberculosis

A 44-year-old male, refugee living in a camp, with weight loss, fever, and productive cough, presenting to the ED. A chest radiograph was requested, depicting apical opacities with cavitation. Immediately after this, a chest CT scan is ordered by the emergency physician for "better clarification." Meanwhile, ED lab results are ready, revealing acid-fast bacilli (AFB) on sputum examination.

## 5.1 Role of Imaging: A Value-Based Approach

Chest radiograph is the first recommended imaging exam in patients with suspected active tuberculosis (TB) (including cavitary form, the so-called open TB), being rated 9 on the 9-point scale of the ACR Appropriateness Criteria (2018). In the same guideline, chest CT comes in second place (rated 7): reasonable to order if CXR is equivocal.

A positive nucleic acid amplification (NAA) test, which can be available within hours, is considered sufficient for the initial diagnosis of tuberculosis, as stated on most recent ATS/Infectious Diseases Society of America (IDSA)/Centers for Disease Control and Prevention (CDCP) practice guidelines on the diagnosis of tuberculosis (Lewinsohn et al. 2017).

---

- **TB disease**: Symptoms and signs of disease in individuals infected with *Mycobacterium tuberculosis*; a positive NAA test (with or without AFB smear positivity) is considered sufficient for initial diagnosis (Lewinsohn et al. 2017).
- **The added value of NAA test**: The sensitivity of AFB examination might not be that high (45–80%), but NAA testing in TB patients with *negative smears* reaches values as high as 80% (Centers for Disease Control and Prevention (CDC) 2009). If the NAA result is negative, it is recommended to test an additional specimen and test for inhibitors (Centers for Disease Control and Prevention (CDC) 2009).
- **Latent tuberculosis infection (LTBI)**: Infected individuals that present no clinical evidence of disease; interferon-γ release assay (IGRA) or tuberculin skin test (TST) are the mainstay for testing (Lewinsohn et al. 2017).

In computed tomography, the pattern of tree in bud or cellular bronchiolitis is certainly not pathognomonic of tuberculosis. It can indeed be very suggestive in the appropriate clinical setting—which is key for the differential diagnosis—but it is very nonspecific as it can be seen in a myriad of infectious conditions, autoimmune, inflammatory, and neoplastic diseases.

Even in the scenario where AFB smear is negative, but the clinical and radiographic picture is positive, e.g., fever, cough with sputum, consumption, cavitation, or air space opacities in CXR, a positive NAA test can be used as evidence of TB disease. Such strategy, advocated by ATS/IDSA/CDCP, is totally congruent with the fact that no single mention to computed tomography is made throughout that entire guideline on TB diagnosis (Lewinsohn et al. 2017), in keeping with a valuable reduced-radiation diagnostic pathway for the (frequently young) patient with TB disease.

Indeed, the main focus is nowadays to rely on the laboratorial diagnosis, in an era when one does not need to wait for weeks until the culture diagnosis (Lewinsohn et al. 2017; Centers for Disease Control and Prevention (CDC) 2009). Also, in the vast majority of times TB is not an emergent diagnosis. It can be calmly and confidently confirmed within hours with this new generation of genetic lab tests.

Regarding the treatment, the conjoined task force (ATS/IDSA/CDCP) guideline on TB treatment (Nahid et al. 2016) only mentions CXR, stating that it should be considered at:

- Baseline for all patients.
- The second month of treatment if baseline cultures are negative (in patient showing positive cultures at baseline diagnosis, it is not essential).
- The end of treatment if baseline cultures are negative (optional if positive).

Again CT should only be required if diagnosis is inconclusive, or more information about extent, severity, or complications is required that will clearly change the management. CT has been known for a long time to be able to detect subtle changes, such as small foci of cavitation, that might go undetected on CXR. Nevertheless, current ATS/IDSA/CDCP guideline (2016) states that CXR findings are sufficient to decide for the different management (length of treatment) of these two forms of TB disease (cavitary vs. no cavitary) (Nahid et al. 2016).

The concern of active airborne spreading of TB should logically be set on a patient with main respiratory complaints (namely cough) who is found to have AFB or a positive NAA test on sputum. Not to be confused, the miliary pattern of TB on CXR means hematogenous dissemination, in a patient whose main complaints are not respiratory and with the main focus of TB being non-pulmonary. Chest CT can also be helpful for better depicting pleuroparenchymal or airway late complications or sequela, e.g., fibronodular scarring and bronchiectasis.

Even a computer software seems to be capable to detect TB on CXR with an area under the curve of 0.99 (Lakhani and Sundaram 2017). This could be very valuable in underdeveloped or remote areas lacking access to radiology expertise or expensive imaging. On the other hand, in some practices, like in Germany, where TB is not endemic, more emphasis is sometimes put on chest CT due to lack of expertise in TB CXR reading or of awareness by the requesting physicians. Often, it is in a context of a "fever of unknown origin; extensive lab workup negative" that the radiologist—while reading the CT scan—is the first to suggest this diagnosis and to point towards the missing lab tests not yet ordered.

**Key Points**
- **Appropriateness of request**: CXR is most of the times the sufficient imaging test of choice for baseline workup of TB disease, and for subsequent follow-up at 2 months and end of treatment (mainly if baseline cultures are negative, in these two last time points).
- **Increase value, reduce radiation, reduce costs**: For the initial diagnostic workup, chest CT should be reserved for the cases in which a CXR may be negative or equivocal for active and/or open TB, there is a high suspicion or the patient is clearly symptomatic, but the laboratorial tests are inconclusive.

# 6    Case 5: Acute Respiratory Illness (ARI)

A 33-year-old male with inflammatory bowel disease (IBD) is treated in an ambulatory setting with a drug known to have a risk of tuberculosis reactivation/development as a possible side effect: infliximab. He presents to the ED with fever (39.5 °C) and altered mental status. A head CT scan showed some ring-enhancing lesions compatible with tuberculomas, given the clinical setting. A chest radiograph was also ordered depicting a miliary pattern. Given the immuno-compromised setting and high fever, the ED physician decides to consult the CDS tool (namely the *ARI in Immunocompromised Patients* link option) and requests a chest CT.

## 6.1    Role of Imaging: A Value-Based Approach

In case of acute respiratory illness (ARI), most likely to be related to a noncardiac etiology, one

must first reflect the immune status of the patient, either being immunocompetent or immunocompromised.

### 6.1.1    ARI in Immunocompetent Patients

The ACR Appropriateness Criteria defines nine possible variants (American College of Radiology Appropriateness Criteria® 2018). Briefly, they are summarized as exacerbation of asthma or COPD (complicated vs. uncomplicated, in each setting), patient >40 years old, patient <40 years old (with vs. without risk factors or signs), patient with dementia (any age), and complicated pneumonia. For all these variants, the most appropriate and high-rated exam is CXR (American College of Radiology Appropriateness Criteria® 2018).

For uncomplicated asthma, uncomplicated COPD, and low-risk patients younger than 40 years old, even the indication for a CXR might be questioned. A CT is clearly low rated and not appropriate. This is in concordance with most recent British Thoracic Society (BTS) guideline on community-acquired pneumonia (CAP) who states that it is not even necessary to perform a CXR in all patients with suspected CAP (Lim et al. 2009). In a more conservative approach, IDSA/ATS state that a CXR should be obtained whenever CAP is suspected in adults to establish or rule out the diagnosis, complications, or alternative diagnoses (Mandell et al. 2007).

### 6.1.2    ARI in Immunocompromised Patients

The ACR only defines four possible variants (American College of Radiology Appropriateness Criteria® 2018). CXR is also the initial exam to be considered, and depending on the results of this initial step—negative, equivocal, nonspecific, or positive CXR—a chest CT without contrast could also be considered, if it alters the management or gives valuable additional information. Evidence of early invasive pulmonary aspergillosis in febrile patients submitted to stem cell transplantation, when CXRs are sometimes initially negative, is a good example. In cases where CXR shows scattered opacities, the ability of CT to detect halos of ground glass opacity around such opacities, again in febrile patients submitted to stem cell transplantation, is another good example for the early presumptive diagnosis of invasive aspergillosis that strongly supports the initiation of empiric antifungal therapy.

Cytomegalovirus and *Pneumocystis jirovecii* pneumonias are further examples, where one can face a CXR positive for atypical pneumonia, but the CT patterns will provide additional valuable clues if taken together with the precise clinical setting. Frequently, CXR will be negative or inconclusive, while CT will clearly show patterns of atypical pneumonia.

This case scenario however illustrates how pure reliance on CDS tools can be tricky or misleading. Based on a positive CXR depicting a miliary pattern in an immunocompromised patient, one could simply click on the options inside the "*ARI in Immunocompromised*

*Patients*" and figure out that in case of a "positive chest radiograph" a chest CT would be rated as appropriate. But as we have seen on the previous case scenario about tuberculosis, a chest CT would only be appropriate in equivocal cases. ACR Appropriateness Criteria has a separate link for "*Imaging of possible TB*," which makes sense as this is a special and rather specific type of pneumonia (American College of Radiology Appropriateness Criteria® 2018).

Our case scenario of a young adult with IBD taking infliximab, fever, positive head CT, and a miliary pattern on CXR is straightforward (not equivocal) for a reactivation or development of TB with hematogenous spread. Thus, in this scenario the chest CT can be regarded as inappropriate (Fig. 2).

Imaging investigation of acute dyspnea with a suspected cardiac origin should also be started with CXR before additional exams, CXR being in all the cardiac scenarios once again top rated by ACR (American College of Radiology Appropriateness Criteria® 2018). This will be explained in more detail in another chapter in this book.

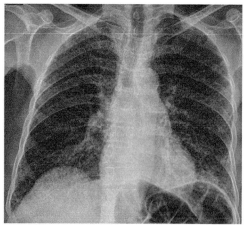 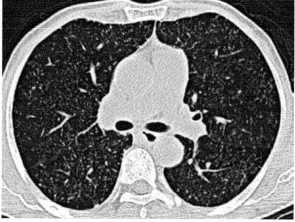

**Fig. 2** Chest radiograph and CT showing a miliary pattern. On CT the random micronodule distribution is clearly depicted. Images are from a companion case [reprinted by permission from Springer Nature: Carrillo-Bayona J.A., Arias-Alvarez L. (2018) Diagnostic Imaging in Sepsis of Pulmonary Origin. In: Ortiz-Ruiz G., Dueñas-Castell C. (eds) Sepsis. Springer, New York, NY (DOI: https://doi.org/10.1007/978-1-4939-7334-7_5)]

**Key Points**

- **Appropriateness of request**: Chest radiograph is the first choice to be considered in immunocompetent patients, in all listed possible variants for ARI, being the most appropriate and high-rated exam (American College of Radiology Appropriateness Criteria® 2018).

  For immunocompromised patients, after an initial CXR, chest CT is appropriate (e.g., aspergillosis in stem cell-transplanted patient).

- **Patient-centered care**: The sole reliance on CDS tools might be misleading. Chest CT as a second-line or problem-solving exam for specific ARI etiologies should be used judiciously, preferably after multidisciplinary discussion with a radiologist.

## 7    Case 6: Blunt Trauma … and a Mediastinal Mass

A chest CT is requested for a 39-year-old female who had blunt trauma after a motor vehicle accident. In the requesting form, there was no information with regard to speed or acceleration/deceleration details. The CT was done, and no thoracic evidence of trauma was depicted, but an incidental, nonspecific, regularly shaped mass was found in the anterior mediastinum.

## 7.1    Role of Imaging: A Value-Based Approach

CXR and chest CT with contrast/CT angiography are top rated and regarded as complementary first-line imaging exams in the initial workup of patients with high-energy blunt thoracic trauma, as per current ACR Appropriateness Criteria

(2018). In case of non-high-energy mechanism and after a careful trauma survey reveals very low probability of significant thoracic trauma, further assessment with chest CT(A) may not be necessary. Bottom line, the decision to order a CT in this setting is somewhat subjective as it depends on the information about the mechanism of the trauma and is prone to significant variance in local practices.

### 7.1.1    What Constitutes a High-Energy Mechanism? When to Safely Forego a CT?

In a recently published landmark paper (2015), decision instruments were prospectively validated and shown to identify clinically significant blunt thoracic trauma (in patients aged older than 14 years) and to help avoid CT in nearly a third of people admitted to ED, without increasing the risk of missing major injury (Rodriguez et al. 2015). Known as "NEXUS Chest CT," this decision instrument consists of a set of criteria, namely:

- Abnormal CXR (any thoracic injury—including clavicle fracture—or a widened mediastinum).
- Distracting injury (such as a broken thigh bone).
- Tenderness in the chest wall, sternum, scapula, or thoracic spine.
- Injury caused by rapid deceleration—either a fall of >20 ft (6.1 m) or a motor vehicle accident while travelling >40 mph (64.4 km/h).

The application of these criteria, to sort out who can't and who can safely forego a chest CT, should be considered for a local and institution-approved practice, if one wants to reduce the number of negative CT scans, cost, radiation exposure, or implications from incidentalomas.

As CDS tools for imaging exams are in their inception, and the main brands rely heavily on ACR Appropriateness Criteria and because for some specific topics they might be not up-to-date, one must use them with a critical reasoning.

### 7.1.2   What About the Incidentaloma (Mediastinal Mass) in This Young Patient?

The negative chest CT for trauma injuries depicted a regular mass in the anterior mediastinum. Differential diagnosis would include, for example, thymoma, lymphoma, thymic cyst, or thymic hyperplasia. Nevertheless, the diagnosis relying solely on the CT images from the trauma protocol can sometimes be impossible.

Bipyramidal morphology and presence of gross intercalated fat (aspects said to be pathognomonic) are present on CT imaging in only about half of cases for thymic hyperplasia (Ackman et al. 2015). Frequently, when in favor of a possible or most likely diagnosis of thymoma, surgical resection is the next step, as CT-guided biopsy for thymoma is discouraged due to the capsule nature of the mass and risk of seeding. Thus, in many instances thymectomies will be performed, which turn out to be unnecessary. In some studies the frequency is estimated to range from 28% to 44% (Ackman et al. 2015; Kent et al. 2014).

Further preoperative diagnostic workup using MRI can be really helpful to reduce these thymectomies. MRI of the chest with in-phase and out-of-phase sequences can distinguish thymic hyperplasia, which presents with a signal drop, from thymic neoplasm or lymphoma, which does not show a signal drop (Priola et al. 2015). MRI can also better depict the cystic nature of a lesion with T2-weighted sequences, being considered the first step in the management of incidental nonspecific mass lesions found on thoracic CT exams by the ACR Committee on Incidental Findings (Munden et al. 2018). In the few cases where a normal thymus or hyperplasia does not exhibit a signal drop (Fig. 3), DWI can be helpful in at least ruling out lymphoma in patients younger than 30 years (Priola et al. 2018).

Table 2 briefly summarizes the main MRI features of these different mediastinal masses.

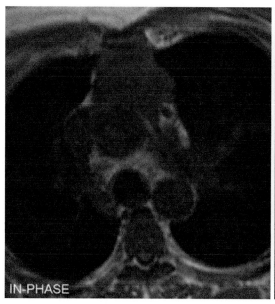

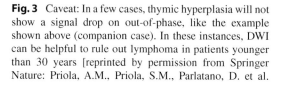

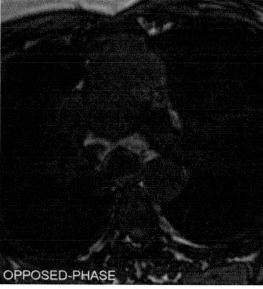

**Fig. 3** Caveat: In a few cases, thymic hyperplasia will not show a signal drop on out-of-phase, like the example shown above (companion case). In these instances, DWI can be helpful to rule out lymphoma in patients younger than 30 years [reprinted by permission from Springer Nature: Priola, A.M., Priola, S.M., Parlatano, D. et al. Apparent diffusion coefficient measurements in diffusion-weighted magnetic resonance imaging of the anterior mediastinum: inter-observer reproducibility of five different methods of region-of-interest positioning. Eur Radiol (2017) 27: 1386. (DOI: https://doi.org/10.1007/s00330-016-4527-8)]

**Key Points**

- **Increase value, reduce costs, reduce radiation**: NEXUS Chest CT decision instrument allows a safe reduction of approximately 25–37% of unnecessary chest CTs in the setting of blunt trauma (Rodriguez et al. 2015).
- **Value of MRI in mediastinal masses**: Once a mediastinal mass is incidentally detected, signal drop on out-of-phase in dual-echo MRI can diagnose a normal thymus or thymic hyperplasia, helping to avoid an unnecessary thymectomy. In some equivocal cases, DWI can further clarify, if a lymphoma or a nonneoplastic cyst is the most likely differential diagnosis.

**Table 2** Typical MRI features of common mediastinal mass lesions

| Mediastinal mass lesion | MRI features |
| --- | --- |
| Thymic hyperplasia | The vast majority suppresses on out-of-phase imaging. |
| Thymoma | Do not suppress on out-of-phase imaging. |
| Lymphoma | Do not suppress on out-of-phase imaging. Lower ADC values on DWI comparatively to thymic hyperplasia on patients <30 years old (Priola et al. 2018). |
| Nonneoplastic cyst | Usually a typical high T2 signal and lack of enhancement. The high ADC values in cysts more accurately distinguish them from solid masses with equivocal enhancement or T2 signal (Shin et al. 2014). |

## 8    Case 7: Cancer Staging and Follow-Up: The Best Protocol

A contrast-enhanced CT scan of the thorax and abdomen was requested for a 62-year-old male, who is on follow-up for his treated lung cancer. The patient asks if this exam is going to have multiple steps of breath-holding, as he felt some-what uncomfortable some time ago when he was submitted for an abdominal CT scan (liver lesion protocol with four phases). Also, he asks if it is really necessary to fast, as he is somewhat frail.

## 8.1    Role of Imaging: A Value-Based Approach

Contrast-enhanced CT of the chest and upper abdomen has a pivotal role in the initial staging workup and follow-up of thoracic malignancies, especially lung cancer.

### 8.1.1    One or Two Acquisitions: What's Best?

When in charge for a CT scan protocol, a frequent dilemma the attending radiologist faces is to consider one single acquisition (60-s delay) or two acquisitions (35-s delay for thorax, plus 70-s delay for abdomen). Previous literature regarding this issue seemed somewhat sparse or conflicting. Interestingly, a recent randomized controlled crossover clinical trial (García-Garrigós et al. 2018) found that, in patients with lung cancer, a single (60-s delayed acquisition for thorax and abdomen) was associated with less contrast artifact, afforded better visualization of lymph nodes, and had lower radiation dose while maintaining acceptable vascular and hepatic enhancement (Fig. 4).

The results from this trial are in concordance also with recent published literature on pleural malignancies that states a particularly lower sensitivity for detection of pleural malignancy when using CT pulmonary angiography (Tsim et al. 2017). Indeed, Tsim et al. have recently retrospectively reviewed 315 patients from the DIAPHRAGM study (a prospective, multicenter observational study of mesothelioma biomarkers) to assess the diagnostic performance of CT in suspected pleural malignancy. They found that almost half of the patients with pleural malignancy had a benign CT report. More importantly, sensitivity in CTPA studies was significantly inferior to that of venous-phase CT (27% vs. 61%; $p = 0.0056$). They also found that sensitivity was lower with non-thoracic radiology reporting (Tsim et al. 2017).

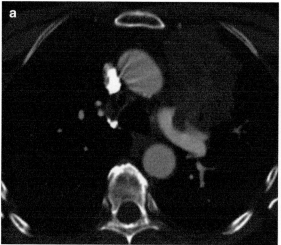 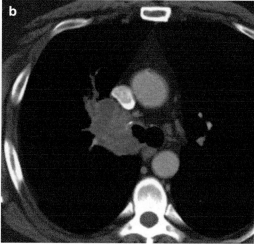

**Fig. 4** Companion case showing contrast artifact in the superior vena cava (**a**). The single acquisition protocol (**b**) is less prone to such artifacts while maintaining acceptable vascular enhancement and better visualization of lymph nodes [reprinted by permission from Springer Nature: Ravenel J.G. (2016) Staging of Lung Cancer. In: Schoepf U., Meinel F. (eds) Multidetector-Row CT of the Thorax. Medical Radiology. Springer, Cham. (DOI: https://doi.org/10.1007/978-3-319-30355-0_11)]

### 8.1.2 To Fast or Not to Fast?

Regarding the issue of fasting—also a topic of some discussion between referrers, patients, and radiologists—a recent landmark study (Barbosa et al. 2018) (prospective and random) found very few adverse symptoms regardless of preparative fasting in cancer patients undergoing contrast-enhanced CT. Patients who fasted were more likely to be dehydrated, irritable, and uncooperative during the imaging examination. These findings are in concordance with guidelines endorsed by the French Radiology Society (CIRTACI Comité Interdisciplinaire de Recherche et de Travail sur les Agents de Contraste en Imagerie 2005).

> **Key Points**
> - **Single acquisition protocols** with a 60-s delay are now more convincingly regarded as the best for imaging of thoracic malignancies, namely lung and pleural cancer and their follow-up.
> - **Fasting**: Fasting before contrast-enhanced CT can be more detrimental, and it does not decrease the likelihood of main adverse reactions.

### 9 Summary

In chest imaging, radiologists can add value to the episode of care through:

- Outcomes improvement, like when suggesting additional imaging exams that can prevent the patient to be submitted to unnecessary harmful and costly surgery (thymectomy avoidance once MRI diagnoses a nonneoplastic mass), or when rising patient satisfaction and safety, e.g., when choosing the best protocol for CT, avoiding harmful fasting, and avoiding unnecessary acquisitions or breath-hold steps that can be hard to cope for the patient.
- Cost reduction, like avoidance of redundant or inappropriate imaging, e.g., daily CXR in the ICU, preoperative radiographs in low-risk stable patients, and chest CT use in clear-cut initial diagnosis of ARDS or TB.

In this way, it is imperative that the entire multidisciplinary team works on the same lane and with the same mindset, to better work in a value-based environment, because only positive inputs from different sides will lead to the maximum gain in value, either through the equation numerator (outcomes) or through the denominator (costs).

# References

Ackman JB, Verzosa S, Kovach AE et al (2015) High rate of unnecessary thymectomy and its cause. Can computed tomography distinguish thymoma, lymphoma, thymic hyperplasia, and thymic cysts? Eur J Radiol 84(3):524–533

American College of Radiology Appropriateness Criteria®. https://www.acr.org/Clinical-Resources/ACR-Appropriateness-Criteria. Accessed 14 Aug 2018

Banks PA, Bollen TL, Dervenis C et al (2013) Classification of acute pancreatitis – 2012: revision of the Atlanta classification and definitions by international consensus. Gut 62:102–111

Barbosa PNVP, Bitencourt AGV, Tyng CJ et al (2018) Preparative fasting for contrast-enhanced CT in a cancer center: a new approach. AJR Am J Roentgenol 210(5):941–947

Centers for Disease Control and Prevention (CDC) (2009) Updated Guidelines for the use of nucleic acid amplification tests in the diagnosis of tuberculosis. MMWR Morb Mortal Wkly Rep 58(1):7–10

Choosing Wisely®. The American Board of Internal Medine Foundation. http://www.choosingwisely.org/wp-content/uploads/2015/01/Choosing-Wisely-Recommendations.pdf. Accessed 14 Aug 2018

CIRTACI Comité Interdisciplinaire de Recherche et de Travail sur les Agents de Contraste en Imagerie. Prescribing fasting before a radiological examination requiring the use of iodinated contrast media. Société Française de Radiologie website. http://www.sfrnet.org/data/upload/files/a7e7222e420ac-736c1256b6c0044cb07/contrast%20media%20pre-scribing%20fasting.pdf. Published 2005. Accessed 14 Aug 2018

Committee on Standards and Practice Parameters (2012) Practice advisory for preanesthesia evaluation: an updated report by the American Society of Anesthesiologists Task Force on Preanesthesia Evaluation. Anesthesiology 116(3):522–538

Danielson D, Bjork K, Card R, Foreman J, Harper C, Roemer R, Stultz J, Sypura W, Thompson S, Webb B. Institute for Clinical Systems Improvement. Health Care Guideline - Preoperative Evaluation. Updated July 2012. http://aspiruslibrary.org/guidelines_new/ICSI%20Preop%20Guideline.pdf. Accessed 14 Aug 2108

den Harder AM, de Heer LM, de Jong PA et al (2018) Frequency of abnormal findings on routine chest radiography before cardiac surgery. J Thorac Cardiovasc Surg 155(5):2035–2040

Fan E, Del Sorbo L, Goligher EC et al (2017) An Official American Thoracic Society/European Society of Intensive Care Medicine/Society of Critical Care Medicine Clinical Practice Guideline: Mechanical Ventilation in Adult Patients with Acute Respiratory Distress Syndrome. Am J Respir Crit Care Med 195(9):1253–1263

Fan E, Brodie D, Slutsky AS (2018) Acute respiratory distress syndrome: advances in diagnosis and treatment. JAMA 319(7):698–710

Ferguson ND, Frutos-Vivar F, Esteban A et al (2005) Acute respiratory distress syndrome: underrecognition by clinicians and diagnostic accuracy of three clinical definitions. Crit Care Med 33(10):2228–2234

Fröhlich S, Murphy N, Doolan A et al (2013) Acute respiratory distress syndrome: under recognition by clinicians. J Crit Care 28(5):663–668

García-Garrigós E, Arenas-Jiménez JJ, Sánchez-Payá J (2018) Best protocol for combined contrast-enhanced thoracic and abdominal CT for lung cancer: a single-institution randomized crossover clinical trial. AJR Am J Roentgenol 210(6):1226–1234

Goodman LR, Fumagalli R, Tagliabue P et al (1999) Adult respiratory distress syndrome due to pulmonary and extrapulmonary causes: CT, clinical, and functional correlations. Radiology 213(2):545–552

Hejblum G, Chalumeau-Lemoine L, Ioos V et al (2009) Comparison of routine and on-demand prescription of chest radiographs in mechanically ventilated adults: a multicentre, cluster-randomised, two-period crossover study. Lancet 374(9702):1687–1693

Joo HS, Wong J, Naik VN, Savoldelli GL (2005) The value of screening preoperative chest x-rays: a systematic review. Can J Anaesth 52:568–574

Kent MS, Wang T, Gangadharan SP, Whyte RI (2014) What is the prevalence of a "nontherapeutic" thymectomy? Ann Thorac Surg 97:276–282, discussion, 282

Keveson B, Clouser RD, Hamlin MP et al (2017) Adding value to daily chest X-rays in the ICU through education, restricted daily orders and indication-based prompting. BMJ Open Qual 6(2):e000072

Lakhal K, Serveaux-Delous M, Lefrant JY, Capdevila X, Jaber S (2012) Chest radiographs in 104 French ICUs: current prescription strategies and clinical value (the RadioDay study). Intensive Care Med 38(11):1787–1799

Lakhani P, Sundaram B (2017) Deep learning at chest radiography: automated classification of pulmonary tuberculosis by using convolutional neural networks. Radiology 284(2):574–582

Lewinsohn DM, Leonard MK, LoBue PA et al (2017) Official American Thoracic Society/Infectious Diseases Society of America/Centers for Disease Control and Prevention Clinical Practice Guidelines: Diagnosis of Tuberculosis in Adults and Children. Clin Infect Dis 64(2):111–115

Lim WS, Baudouin SV, George RC et al (2009) BTS guidelines for the management of community acquired pneumonia in adults: update 2009. Thorax 64:iii1–iii55

Mandell LA, Wunderink RG, Anzueto A et al (2007) Infectious Diseases Society of America/American Thoracic Society consensus guidelines on the management of community-acquired pneumonia in adults. Clin Infect Dis 44(Suppl 2):S27–S72

Munden RF, Carter BW, Chiles C et al (2018) Managing incidental findings on thoracic CT: mediastinal and cardiovascular findings. A white paper of the ACR incidental findings committee. J Am Coll Radiol 15(8):1087–1096

Nahid P, Dorman SE, Alipanah N et al (2016) Official American Thoracic Society/Centers for Disease Control and Prevention/Infectious Diseases Society of America Clinical Practice Guidelines: Treatment of Drug-Susceptible Tuberculosis. Clin Infect Dis 63(7):e147–e195

Oba Y, Zaza T (2010) Abandoning daily routine chest radiography in the intensive care unit: meta-analysis. Radiology 255(2):386–395

Priola AM, Priola SM, Ciccone G et al (2015) Differentiation of rebound and lymphoid thymic hyperplasia from anterior mediastinal tumors with dual-echo chemical-shift MR imaging in adulthood: reliability of the chemical-shift ratio and signal intensity index. Radiology 274(1):238–249

Priola AM, Priola SM, Gned D et al (2018) Nonsuppressing normal thymus on chemical-shift MR imaging and anterior mediastinal lymphoma: differentiation with diffusion-weighted MR imaging by using the apparent diffusion coefficient. Eur Radiol 28(4):1427–1437

Ranieri VM, Rubenfeld GD, Thompson BT, Ferguson ND, Caldwell E, Fan E et al (2012) Acute respiratory distress syndrome: the Berlin definition. JAMA 307:2526–2533

Rodriguez RM, Langdorf MI, Nishijima D et al (2015) Derivation and validation of two decision instruments for selective chest CT in blunt trauma: a multicenter prospective observational study (NEXUS Chest CT). PLoS Med 12(10):e1001883

Shin KE, Yi CA, Kim TS et al (2014) Diffusion-weighted MRI for distinguishing non-neoplastic cysts from solid masses in the mediastinum: problem-solving in mediastinal masses of indeterminate internal characteristics on CT. Eur Radiol 24(3):677–684

Thoeni RF (2015) Imaging of Acute Pancreatitis. Radiol Clin N Am 53(6):1189–1208

Tsim S, Stobo DB, Alexander L, Kelly C, Blyth KG (2017) The diagnostic performance of routinely acquired and reported computed tomography imaging in patients presenting with suspected pleural malignancy. Lung Cancer 103:38–43

Ware LB, Bastarache JA, Bernard GR (2017) Acute respiratory distress syndrome. In: Vincent JL et al (eds) Textbook of critical care, 7th edn. Elsevier, Philadelphia, PA

Zhou MT, Chen CS, Chen BC et al (2010) Acute lung injury and ARDS in acute pancreatitis: mechanisms and potential intervention. World J Gastroenterol 16(17):2094–2099

# Value-Based Radiology in Abdominal and Pelvic Imaging

Kheng L. Lim

## Contents

K. L. Lim (✉)
Department of Radiology, Pennsylvania Hospital,
University of Pennsylvania Health System,
Philadelphia, PA, USA
e-mail: Kheng.Lim@uphs.upenn.edu

**Abstract**

In this chapter, five cases are presented to illustrate the central role of radiologists in patient care. These cases illustrate the incredible value that the radiologists can bring to the table, and the input of radiologists in promoting evidence-based guidelines in the management of patients. Clinical algorithms in determining when an abdominopelvic CT examination is indicated for blunt abdominopelvic trauma are discussed. A case in the workup of incidentalomas shows the potential for high-value care radiologists can offer to patients, a case illustrating the radiologist ability to influence medical versus surgical management of appendicitis in the era where imaging diagnosis has arguably trumped over clinical diagnosis of appendicitis. Cases discussing the central role of radiologists in diagnosing renal colic and colonic diverticulitis, and the potential for radiologists to act as patients advocate to minimize unnecessary radiation exposure associated with CT scans, are also discussed.

## 1 Introduction

In many developed nations, healthcare spending has often outpaced the growth of the gross domestic product (GDP). For example, health spending in the United States is projected to grow 1% point faster than the GDP per year over

Med Radiol Diagn Imaging (2019)
https://doi.org/10.1007/174_2018_204, © Springer Nature Switzerland AG
Published Online: 16 February 2019

**Table 1** Case scenarios to be displayed in this chapter

| Case | Issue | Key points |
|---|---|---|
| Case 1 | When to scan and when not to scan patients presenting with blunt abdominal trauma | Validated clinical algorithms can help clinicians in reducing unnecessary CT scans while increasing diagnostic yield of CT scans |
| Case 2 | Incidental adrenal nodule | Always check for prior studies when an incidentaloma is encountered on imaging. Being aware of practice guidelines from professional societies can be of value in managing patients with incidentalomas |
| Case 3 | Appendicitis—surgical versus medical management | Structured reporting of features associated with complicated appendicitis can improve treatment outcomes of patients |
| Case 4 | CT utilization for recurrent episodes of renal colic | Alternative imaging using ultrasound to assess for hydronephrosis and plain radiography to detect stones can provide similar diagnostic value to CT in patients with acute flank pain and suspected urolithiasis |
| Case 5 | Heavy reliance on imaging to diagnose colonic diverticulitis | CT diagnosis of colonic diverticulitis is the gold standard. Alternative use of ultrasound with graded compression may provide similar diagnostic value in select hands. Discussion on the controversy of colonic malignancy initially manifested as perforated diverticulitis |

the 2017–2026 period. Clearly, this disproportionate growth cannot be sustained. In order to achieve a more efficient delivery of health care, practicing medicine in status quo is now being scrutinized. Healthcare payment will gradually shift from a purely volume-based model to a value-based payment model where good patient outcomes dictate physician and hospital reimbursement. This chapter presents five real cases of diseases and commonly encountered scenarios in the abdomen and pelvis (Table 1), lessons learned from these cases, and discussion of how radiologists can make a difference in achieving better patient outcomes while reducing healthcare cost.

## 2 Case 1 Blunt Abdominal Trauma

Sixty-eight-Year-old female with 2-week history of intermittent vertigo presented to the emergency department (ED) after a fall from getting off the bed in the middle of the night, hitting an end table, and developed pain over the right lower ribs and flank. Physical examination reported skin abrasion without open wound, tender to palpation of right lateral lower ribs, and Glasgow Coma Scale of 15. The patient's vital

signs were stable with mildly elevated blood pressure of 141/75 mmHg, pulse of 84, and respiratory rate of 20.

The patient's past medical history was significant for hyperlipidemia, non-active hyperparathyroidism, diabetes, asthma, and obstructive sleep apnea. There was no history of being on anticoagulation or congestive heart failure. The patient had a normal hematologic profile.

The clinician in the ED ordered a computed tomography (CT) of the head, thorax, abdomen, and pelvis to assess for trauma-related injuries.

*CT scan results*: No acute intracranial abnormality was detected on the head CT (not shown). The thoracic and abdominopelvic CT was only significant for mild subcutaneous fat stranding in the right flank, reflecting traumatic changes from blunt contusion (Fig. 1).

### 2.1 Role of Imaging: A Value-Based Approach

Blunt trauma resulting in physical pain commonly drives patients to seek medical attention and the most accessible medical consultation is at an emergency department of a hospital. CT scan is a powerful tool in diagnosing clinically significant, trauma-related injuries. Because

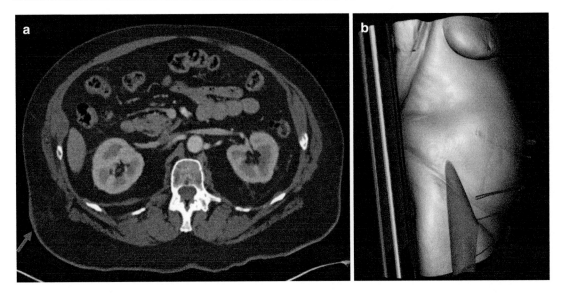

**Fig. 1** Axial CT image (**a**) shows subtle stranding of the right flank subcutaneous tissue (arrow). 3D reconstructed surface view (**b**) of the right side of the torso shows no penetrating wound

CT scanner is readily available in a hospital setting, it is often utilized in aiding clinical triaging and medical decision-making. Every patient who presents with trauma can often be appropriately triaged if the patient undergoes a CT scan but this is obviously not an effective use of CT scan. The clinician should weigh the risks and benefits of a CT diagnosis including radiation exposure, cost, and incidentalomas and their downstream costs and risks of further workup.

Baghdanian et al. presented an algorithm implemented at their institution (level 1 trauma hospital in Boston, USA) to help the clinicians triage patients presenting with blunt abdominopelvic trauma (BAPT) (Baghdanian et al. 2017). Their study showed that their institution was able to reduce the number of CT scans performed (a decrease of 32% from pre-intervention to post-intervention period) while increasing the number of significant positive CT findings for BAPT (12.3–17.5%). Also, a significant decrease in hospital length of stay but without any increase in patient mortality was shown. Their clinical algorithm starts first with assessment of:

– Systolic blood pressure (SBP) >90 mmHg?
– Glasgow Coma Scale ≥11?

An exploratory pathway (clinical judgment by the surgeon if laparotomy is necessary) is considered if the first question is negative (i.e., SBP ≤90 mmHg), and an immediate abdominopelvic CT scan is ordered if the patient is not hemodynamically unstable but the second question turns out to be negative, as intoxication or other trauma-related issues often result in an inaccurate history or physical examination.

If both questions are positive, then physical examination of the chest and abdomen, assessment for gross hematuria, and assessment for pelvic, humeral, thigh, and leg fractures are done. If positive, an abdominopelvic CT scan should be considered. If negative, further assessment of risk factors and comorbidities such as anticoagulation, hemodialysis, heart failure, thrombocytopenia, and cirrhosis is taken to determine whether to admit the patient for observation or safe discharge.

Better imaging utilization can be achieved with the case example presented above. Instead of ordering a CT of the thorax, ordering a PA and lateral radiographs of the thorax with or without rib radiographs appear equivalent in rendering clinically significant diagnosis (Rodriguez et al. 2013). After all, the symptoms in our patient were localized to the junction of the thorax and abdomen which could be assessed on the CT of the abdomen covering the lower portion of the thorax.

> **Key Points**
> - **Appropriate request:** Clinical algorithms can be implemented to help guide clinicians in determining when an abdominopelvic CT examination is indicated for blunt abdominopelvic trauma. An institution-approved algorithm can also provide a foundation for the clinicians to stand on when malpractice accusations are brought against them by the patients.
> - **Increase value, reduce radiation:** Clinical algorithms can be used to reduce the use of CT in the emergency department by preventing unnecessary CT scans when the patients meet predetermined, clinically based criteria.

## 3    Case 2: Adrenal Mass

Fifty-one-Year-old male presented to a hospital ED complaining of left-sided chest and abdominal pain after a fall off a ladder 2 days prior to presentation. The patient's past medical history was only significant for hypertension and mild asthma. A CT of the thorax, abdomen, and pelvis was performed to evaluate for internal trauma.

No acute traumatic injury was visualized on the CT of the chest, abdomen, and pelvis. However, an incidental "2.5 cm low-attenuation mass in the right adrenal gland" was noted. The interpreting radiologist stated that "a non-contrast

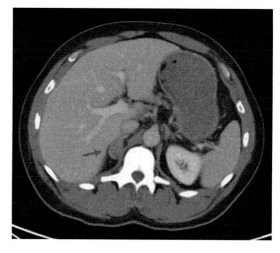

**Fig. 2** Routine axial contrast-enhanced CT image shows an indeterminate right adrenal mass (arrow)

CT of the abdomen could be performed to confirm an adrenal adenoma" (Fig. 2).

The patient read the CT report and was concerned about the incidental adrenal mass. A CT of the abdomen without and with intravenous contrast was subsequently performed 4 months later (Fig. 3).

Unbeknownst to the radiologist recommending further workup of the adrenal mass, the patient had prior CTs performed 6 years prior and 12 years prior (Fig. 4), showing the right adrenal mass.

In this case, further workup with three-phase CT using adrenal mass protocol was unnecessary if the interpreting radiologist had not overlooked the prior CTs. The ability to detect a mass is great but the radiologist would have done an incredible job with the added value of providing a diagnosis based on the knowledge that the adrenal mass presence on the prior CTs reflects a benign, clinically insignificant process. The right adrenal mass had been present for over 10 years and was consistent with a benign adenoma. Further workup with a three-phase CT using adrenal mass protocol is not only unnecessary but can also be harmful for the unnecessary exposure to ionizing radiation.

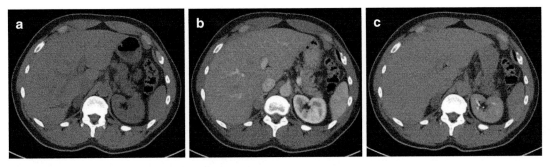

**Fig. 3** (**a**) Axial unenhanced CT shows low-attenuating mass in the right adrenal gland (arrow). (**b**) Axial enhanced CT image shows enhancement of the right adrenal mass.

(**c**) Axial 15-min-delayed enhanced CT image shows >60% absolute washout of the right adrenal adenoma

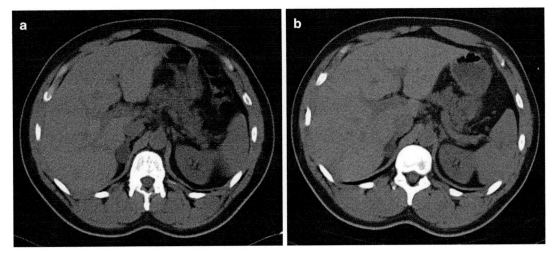

**Fig. 4** (**a**) Axial unenhanced CT image performed 6 years prior shows a low-attenuating right adrenal adenoma with Hounsfield units less than 10 (arrow). (**b**) Axial CT image

performed 12 years prior shows a smaller right adrenal adenoma

## 3.1 Rationale

Adrenal adenoma can be diagnosed on an unenhanced CT scan if the Hounsfield units (HU) are 10 or less (Caoili et al. 2002; Mayo-Smith et al. 2017). There are no added benefits of injecting iodinated contrast intravenously if an adenoma is rich in lipid and has attenuation of 10 HU or less (Mayo-Smith et al. 2017). Therefore, the radiologists can provide added benefits by checking the unenhanced CT

images before deciding on intravenous contrast administration when working up an adrenal mass.

*Caveat*: The relative and absolute washout criteria for the diagnosis of a lipid-poor adenoma overlap with hyper-enhancing lesions such as a pheochromocytoma, renal cell carcinoma metastasis, and hepatocellular carcinoma metastasis (Choi et al. 2013; Patel et al. 2013). Therefore, in these settings, one has to exercise caution of diagnosing a lipid-poor adenoma using the washout criteria (Choi et al. 2013; Patel et al. 2013).

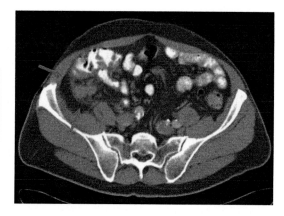

**Fig. 5** Axial CT image shows an amorphous appendix with peri-appendiceal fat stranding (arrows)

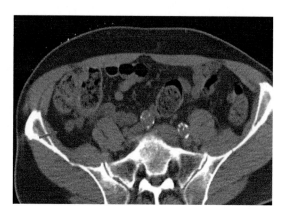

**Fig. 6** Axial CT image from aborted biopsy of cecal "mass" shows improvement of the peri-appendiceal fat stranding

## 4    Case 3: Appendicitis

Seventy-four-Year-old male with untreated chronic lymphocytic leukemia presented to his internist with right lower quadrant abdominal pain for 5 days, which was dull at rest and worse with movement. The working clinical diagnosis was a right inguinal hernia and a CT scan of the abdomen and pelvis was ordered and performed a few days later.

The interpreting radiologist unfortunately concluded that the patient had a mass in the cecum suggestive of colonic malignancy (Fig. 5).

The patient subsequently had a colonoscopy 8 days after the CT, which was reported to be normal. The patient was then referred for an image-guided biopsy of the cecal "mass" a month after the CT but this was not performed as the interventional radiologist could not visualize the "mass" (Fig. 6).

A CT performed 4 months later correctly diagnosed that the perceived cecal "mass" was indeed appendicitis which had essentially resolved (Fig. 7a). A CT scan performed 8 months after the first CT showed that the appendix had normalized (Fig. 7b). The appendix remained present on the CT performed 5 years later (not shown), reflecting complete resolution of the presumed uncomplicated appendicitis.

### 4.1    Role of Imaging: How Can a Structured and Accurate CT Report Help?

This case illustrates the unintended conservative management of uncomplicated appendicitis with spontaneous resolution even without antibiotic therapy. A randomized clinical trial published in

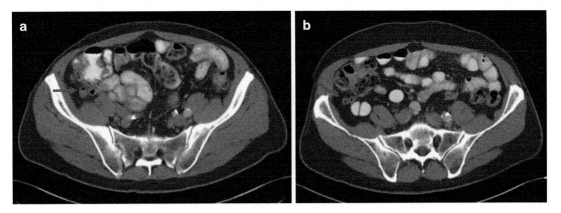

**Fig. 7** (**a**) Axial CT performed 4 months after Fig. 5 shows resolution of the peri-appendiceal fat stranding (arrow). (**b**) CT performed 8 months later after Fig. 5 shows normalization of the appendix

JAMA in 2015 reported that antibiotic therapy could be an option for uncomplicated acute appendicitis (Salminen et al. 2015), which goes along with the argument that some authors use stating that complicated and uncomplicated appendicitis are two discrete entities with differing pathophysiologies (Livingston et al. 2007).

The question in guiding clinical management lies in what should be considered an uncomplicated from complicated appendicitis. Refinements in what should be considered a clear-cut uncomplicated acute appendicitis by imaging, namely CT, are expected in the near future to definitively eliminate concerns about the non-inferior management of such appendicitis with antibiotic therapy. In this regard, a recent systematic review and meta-analysis by Kim et al. (2017) reported that there are nine CT features which can be used for differentiating complicated from uncomplicated appendicitis. These features are as follows:

- Peri-appendiceal fluid collection, abscess, and extraluminal air.
- Appendiceal wall enhancement defect, ascites and ileus.
- Intraluminal air, extraluminal appendicolith, and intraluminal appendicolith.

The CT detection of any of these specific features could be regarded as a predictor for complicated appendicitis that is not amenable to routine antibiotic therapy (Kim et al. 2017).

> **Key Points**
> - **Structured CT report:** Incorporating the presence or absence of these nine CT features can improve communication with the referring surgeon and better assist in the decision of whether or not to choose a conservative strategy for appendicitis.
> - **Increase value, improve outcomes, reduce costs:** Specific CT features to differentiate more confidently complicated from uncomplicated appendicitis are pivotal for cost reduction (unnecessary surgery avoidance) as there is an increasing amount of evidence supporting antibiotic therapy instead of surgery for treating uncomplicated acute appendicitis.

## 5 Case 4: Renal Obstruction from Ureteral Calculi

Thirty-one-Year-old female with a history of kidney stones presented to the ED with left flank pain. She had presented to the same ED within the past month during which a CT performed at that time (Fig. 8) diagnosed her right flank pain secondary to a 4 mm obstructing calculus at the right ureterovesical junction. For this ED presentation, a CT of the abdomen and pelvis was again ordered and performed (Fig. 9). Urinalysis and clinical picture were not consistent with urinary tract infection (UTI).

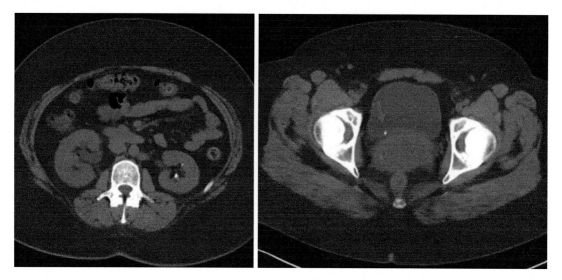

**Fig. 8** Unenhanced axial CT images performed within a month prior to current ED visit shows right hydronephrosis from a 4 mm calculus at the right ureterovesical junction (arrow). Urolithiasis in left kidney was also depicted

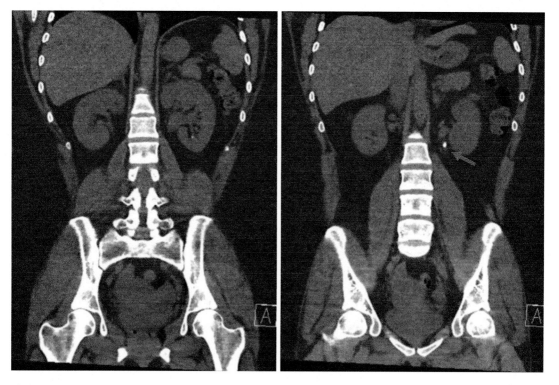

**Fig. 9** Unenhanced coronal CT images show mild left hydronephrosis and proximal hydroureter secondary to a 7 mm proximal left ureteral calculus (arrow)

## 5.1 Role of Imaging: A Value-Based Approach

CT is a powerful tool in rendering accurate diagnosis of obstructive uropathy from calculi lodged in the ureters. However, CT scans should be used judiciously per the ALARA (as low as reasonably achievable) principle on radiation safety (Cohen 2015). This patient had known renal stone disease, presented to the ED with renal colic within the past month, and had a CT showing renal and ureteral calculi. At the second ED presentation, the clinician should be able to reason that the acute left flank pain may be secondary to renal obstruction from ureteral calculi in the absence of UTI. Renal ultrasound (US) is an alternative tool to diagnose hydronephrosis and possibly visualize an obstructing calculus. In a patient with recurrent symptoms from stone disease, it may be excessive to solely rely on CT to diagnose every episode of flank pain without first fully assessing the patient history, clinical presentation, and laboratory data (Turk et al. 2018).

CT is the most accurate imaging modality in the diagnosis of ureteral calculi in patients suspected of renal colic. However, there are downsides of performing a CT, namely radiation exposure and further workup of asymptomatic incidental findings and overcalls.

If hydronephrosis is absent on US, an ensuing CT is likely of low yield to diagnose an obstructing ureteral calculus as the explanation for acute flank pain.

Ripollés et al. reported that CT is the most accurate technique for the detection of ureteral lithiasis; however, the combination of plain radiograph and US is an alternative with good practical value in the setting of acute flank pain (Ripollés et al. 2004).

> **Key Points**
> - **Value of ultrasound:** If imaging is desired, consider ultrasound as a screening and diagnostic tool in patients suspected of renal colic

(Smith-Bindman et al. 2014). The benefits of ultrasound over CT are that ultrasound has no radiation exposure, widespread availability, good reproducibility, and reduced cost relative to CT and is not associated with increased complications or serious adverse events compared to the initial evaluation with CT (Smith-Bindman et al. 2014; Nicolau et al. 2015; Wong et al. 2018).

- **Value of abdominal radiography combined with US:** This may be able to diagnose clinically significant stones; this option should be pursued especially in young patients and those with known stone disease, as stated on current ACR Appropriateness Criteria (Moreno et al. 2018).
- **Value of low-dose CT:** Alternatively, a low-dose non-contrast CT (effective radiation dose <3 mSv which corresponds to about four abdominal radiographs) can be performed in the setting of acute flank pain and suspected ureteral stone (Moreno et al. 2018).

## 6 Case 5: Colonic Diverticulitis

Sixty-three-Year-old female presented to the ED with left-sided abdominal pain with a duration of 2 days, nausea, and subjective fever. She denied diarrhea and blood in the stool. The patient had leukocytosis with $14 \times 10^{12}$/L white blood cells. A CT of the abdomen and pelvis was ordered and the radiologist diagnosed the patient as having diverticulitis involving the distal descending colon with possible intramural abscess (Fig. 10).

The patient was admitted to the inpatient floor for conservative treatment and discharged 3 days later with oral antibiotics. A follow-up CT of the abdomen and pelvis was performed 1.5 months later (Fig. 11). At the time of follow-up CT, the patient was asymptomatic without recurrent pain. The patient had partial colectomy 2 months subsequent to the follow-up CT. Surgical pathology revealed diverticulosis and no malignancy.

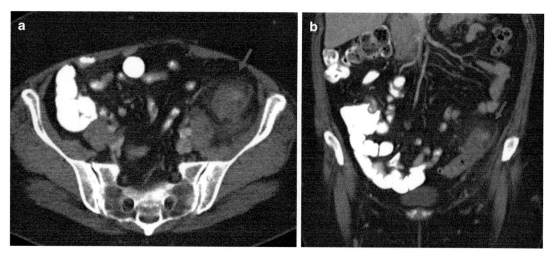

**Fig. 10** (**a**) Axial CT shows peri-colonic stranding surrounding an inflamed diverticulum in the distal descending colon (arrow). No definite abscess or other evidence of colonic macroperforation. (**b**) Coronal CT shows peri-colonic stranding surrounding an inflamed diverticulum in the distal descending colon (arrow)

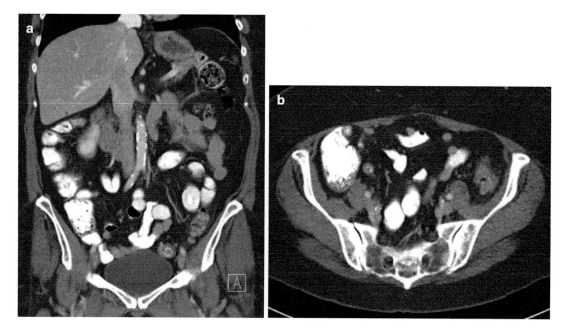

**Fig. 11** (**a**) Coronal CT shows resolution of the distal descending colon diverticulitis. (**b**) Axial CT shows resolution of the distal descending colon diverticulitis

## 6.1 Role of Imaging: When and What?

CT is the most preferred modality in the workup of patients presenting with acute left lower quadrant pain and suspected diverticulitis (McNamara et al. 2018), although a step-up approach with CT performed after an inconclusive or a negative ultrasound (US) is also regarded as a valuable and safe approach, especially in experienced hands (Sartelli et al. 2016).

Recently released new guidelines on classification and management of acute diverticulitis from the World Society of Emergency Surgery (WSES) (Sartelli et al. 2016) have rated CT and US at the same level (level 1C recommendation) with US being used as the first step as explained above.

The rationale of US adoption in the WSES guidelines was based on the European perspective and experience with US technique. The meta-analysis published by Laméris W et al. (2008)—that showed no statistically significant difference in accuracy between US and CT—was followed more recently (2014) by another systematic review and meta-analysis from the Radboud University Nijmegen Medical Centre group in the Netherlands (Andeweg et al. 2014). Again, the results showed that US and CT are comparable in diagnosing acute diverticulitis, with CT having the advantage of more easily identifying alternative diagnoses (Andeweg et al. 2014).

Furthermore, one must remember that nearly 90% of acute diverticulitis diagnosed is in stage Ia (Laméris et al. 2010), that is, a simple confined peri-colic phlegmon, when using the modified Hinchey classification (Kaiser et al. 2005). Such inflammatory changes are usually depicted with ease on US in experienced hands.

Somewhat similar to acute pancreatitis or community-acquired pneumonia for which diagnosis can sometimes be done without imaging support, some authors even argue that the diagnosis of acute diverticulitis can be made, in a considerable percentage (up to 66%), based on clinical evaluation alone (Andeweg et al. 2014; Laméris et al. 2010). In the setting of a patient with recurrent flares and previous colonoscopy negative for malignancy or a recent CT depicting no other potential causes of symptoms such as urolithiasis and hernias, such diagnostic strategy seems reasonable. Nevertheless, adopting a more conservative approach, WSES states that a clinical diagnosis alone is not sufficiently accurate (level 1C recommendation) (Sartelli et al. 2016).

## 6.2 The Concern of Superimposed Colonic Adenocarcinoma

In clinical practice, a follow-up CT is often performed for complicated colonic diverticulitis. The question is whether scanning of the abdomen is necessary when the disease is only localized to the pelvis, and once signs and symptoms of complicated sigmoid or distal descending colon diverticulitis have improved. Keeping in mind the ALARA principle on radiation safety, it seems reasonable to only scan the pelvis in this cohort of patients with improving or resolved symptoms.

The concern that colonic malignancy may mimic complicated/perforated diverticulitis also drives CT utilization in this setting. Lau et al. reported that the overall prevalence of colorectal cancer among their study cohort within 1 year of CT scan was 2.1% (23 of 1,088 cases) (Lau et al. 2011). They found that an odds of having colorectal cancer was higher in patients with diverticular abscess reported on CT (6.7 times higher), local perforation (4 times higher), and fistula (18 times higher) (Lau et al. 2011). A literature review by Sai et al. reported a prevalence of 2.1% of colorectal cancer in patients with CT diagnosis of acute diverticulitis (Sai et al. 2012). Sai et al. however concluded that there is limited data to support the recommendation to perform colonoscopy after a diagnosis of acute diverticulitis. In their meta-analysis, Sharma et al. concluded that while the risk of malignancy after an episode of acute uncomplicated diverticulitis is low (proportional estimate risk of 0.7%), the patients with complicated diverticulitis have much higher risk of colorectal cancer (proportional estimate risk of 10.8%) (Sharma et al. 2014).

> **Key Points**
> - **Value of CT in the initial diagnosis:** High sensitivity and specificity. Has the advantage of more easily identifying alternative diagnoses in patients with left lower quadrant pain.
> - **Value of ultrasound in the initial diagnosis:** Similar accuracy as CT for acute diverticulitis in experienced hands. No radiation and lower cost.
> - **Follow-up/malignancy concern:** In practicing ALARA principle, if a follow-up CT is desired for complicated sigmoid or distal descending diverticulitis, limiting scan range to the pelvis suffices in patients with improving clinical course. Colonoscopy is suggested after resolution of acute diverticulitis, particularly in patients with complicated/perforated diverticulitis to exclude the misdiagnosis of colonic neoplasm (Stollman et al. 2015).

## 7    Summary

As medical diagnosis becomes more reliant on cross-sectional imaging tools and as clinical information becomes more digitized, the window is wide open for radiologists to actively get involved with the management of diseases. The radiologists can play a central role in the diagnosis, management of incidentalomas, provision of directions through current guidelines, and thereby provision of incredible value to patients. In this chapter, we select a few commonly encountered cases and scenarios to illustrate the radiologist's role in contributing to patient care as management of diseases evolves.

## References

Andeweg CS, Wegdam JA, Groenewoud J et al (2014) Toward an evidence-based step-up approach in diagnosing diverticulitis. Scand J Gastroenterol 49:775–784

Baghdanian AH, Baghdanian AA, Armetta A et al (2017) Effect of an institutional triaging algorithm on the use of multidetector CT for patients with blunt abdominopelvic trauma over an 8-year period. Radiology 282(1):84–91

Caoili EM, Korobkin M, Francis IR et al (2002) Adrenal masses: characterization with combined unenhanced and delayed enhanced CT. Radiology 222(3):629–633

Choi YA, Kim CK, Park BK, Kim B (2013) Evaluation of adrenal metastases from renal cell carcinoma and hepatocellular carcinoma: use of delayed contrast-enhanced CT. Radiology 266(2):514–520

Cohen MD (2015) ALARA, image gently and CT-induced cancer. Pediatr Radiol 45(4):465–470

Kaiser AM, Jiang JK, Lake JP et al (2005) The management of complicated diverticulitis and the role of computed tomography. Am J Gastroenterol 100:910–917

Kim HY, Park JH, Lee YJ, Lee SS, Jeon J-J, Lee KH (2017) Systematic review and meta-analysis of CT features for differentiating complicated and uncomplicated appendicitis. Radiology 287(1):104–115

Laméris W, van Randen A, Bipat S et al (2008) Graded compression ultrasonography and computed tomography in acute colonic diverticulitis: meta-analysis of test accuracy. Eur Radiol 18(11):2498–2511

Laméris W, van Randen A, van Gulik TM et al (2010) A clinical decision rule to establish the diagnosis of acute diverticulitis at the emergency department. Dis Colon Rectum 53(6):896–904

Lau KC, Spilsbury K, Farooque Y et al (2011) Is colonoscopy still mandatory after a CT diagnosis of left-sided diverticulitis: can colorectal cancer be confidently excluded? Dis Colon Rectum 54(10):1265

Livingston EH, Woodward WA, Sarosi GA, Haley RW (2007) Disconnect between incidence of nonperforated and perforated appendicitis: implications for pathophysiology and management. Ann Surg 245(6):886–892

Mayo-Smith WW, Song JH, Boland GL et al (2017) Management of incidental adrenal masses: a white paper of the ACR incidental findings committee. J Am Coll Radiol 14(8):1038–1044

McNamara MM, Lalani T, Camacho MA, et al. (2018) ACR appropriateness criteria® left lower quadrant pain—suspected diverticulitis. American College of Radiology. https://acsearch.acr.org/docs/69356/Narrative/. Accessed 18 Sept 2018

Moreno CC, Beland MD, Goldfarb S, et al. (2018) ACR appropriateness criteria® acute onset flank pain—suspicion of stone disease (urolithiasis). American College of Radiology. https://acsearch.acr.org/docs/69362/Narrative/. Accessed 18 Sept 2018

Nicolau C, Claudon M, Derchi LE et al (2015) Imaging patients with renal colic—consider ultrasound first. Insights Imaging 6(4):441–447

Patel J, Davenport MS, Cohan RH, Caoili EM (2013) Can established CT attenuation and washout criteria for adrenal adenoma accurately exclude pheochromocytoma? Am J Roentgenol 201(1):122–127

Ripollés T, Agramunt M, Errando J, Martínez MJ, Coronel B, Morales M (2004) Suspected ureteral colic: plain film and sonography vs unenhanced helical CT. A prospective study in 66 patients. Eur Radiol 14(1):129–136

Rodriguez RM, Anglin D, Langdorf MI et al (2013) NEXUS chest: validation of a decision instrument for selective chest imaging in blunt trauma. JAMA Surg 148(10):940–946

Sai VF, Velayos F, Neuhaus J, Westphalen AC (2012) Colonoscopy after CT diagnosis of diverticulitis to exclude colon cancer: a systematic literature review. Radiology 263(2):383–390

Salminen P, Paajanen H, Rautio T et al (2015) Antibiotic therapy vs. appendectomy for treatment of uncomplicated acute appendicitis: the APPAC randomized clinical trial. JAMA 313(23):2340–2348

Sartelli M, Catena F, Ansaloni L et al (2016) WSES Guidelines for the management of acute left sided colonic diverticulitis in the emergency setting. World J Emerg Surg 11:37

Sharma PV, Eglinton T, Hider P, Frizelle F (2014) Systematic review and meta-analysis of the role of routine colonic evaluation after radiologically confirmed acute diverticulitis. Ann Surg 259(2):263

Smith-Bindman R, Aubin C, Bailitz J et al (2014) Ultrasonography versus computed tomography for suspected nephrolithiasis. N Engl J Med 371(12):1100–1110

Stollman N, Smalley W, Hirano I et al (2015) American gastroenterological association institute guideline on the management of acute diverticulitis. Gastroenterology 149(7):1944–1949

Turk C, Neisius A, Petrik C, et al. (2018) Urolithiasis. European association of urology. http://uroweb.org/guideline/urolithiasis/#3. Accessed 18 Sept 2018

Wong C, Teitge B, Ross M, Young P, Robertson HL, Lang E (2018) The accuracy and prognostic value of point-of-care ultrasound for nephrolithiasis in the emergency department: a systematic review and meta-analysis. Acad Emerg Med 25(6):684–698

# Value-Based Radiology in MSK Imaging

Catarina Ruivo and Diogo Roriz

## Contents

### Abstract

Musculoskeletal disorders are one of the most common problems in the working adult population, leading to loss of productivity and absence, with an obvious impact on the economic status of a community.

Despite what has been done in the last decades, we recommend a change from cost-based to value-based diagnostic algorithms with patient/pathology-tailored protocols which could ultimately provide major economical and medical benefits.

In this chapter we review the values and limitations of the imaging techniques available for the management of musculoskeletal disorders, by presenting some practical cases in which the appropriate and cost-effective approaches are discussed.

## 1 Introduction: Burden of Musculoskeletal Disorders

Musculoskeletal (MSK) diseases are very prevalent and contribute more than any other group of disorders to functional limitations in the adult population in many countries (Woolf and Plefger 2003). They are a group of diseases with low mortality, but high morbidity, affecting the physical and mental health of the patient and its family. This problem has been recognized by the WHO, endorsing the first decade of the millennium as

C. Ruivo
Division of MSK Imaging, CHUC, Coimbra, Portugal

D. Roriz (✉)
Department of Medical Imaging, CHUC, Coimbra, Portugal
e-mail: djr.radiologia@gmail.com

Med Radiol Diagn Imaging (2019)
https://doi.org/10.1007/174_2019_210, © Springer Nature Switzerland AG
Published Online: 23 April 2019

Bone and Joint Decade 2000–2010 (Woolf 2000). Moreover, they are especially prevalent in the working populations (Widanarko et al. 2012), much contributing to a great economic burden on the society associated with an obvious loss of productivity and absence. They encompass a wide group of pathologies, including inflammatory diseases (rheumatoid arthritis and other inflammatory joint diseases), and degenerative, infectious, traumatic, and occupational disorders. Obesity, alcohol consumption, reduced physical activity, smoking, diet, and sports injuries have been some of the culprits of its rising prevalence.

Furthermore, the broader use of medical imaging techniques in the recent years, namely ultrasound (US) and MRI, has played a part in the escalating costs of their diagnosis. Sharpe et al. (2012) reported a 291% increase in the use of MSK ultrasound in the USA from 2000 to 2009 and a corresponding 158% increase in MSK MRI studies in the same period. Early and appropriate diagnosis should therefore be attained in the most cost-effective way, reducing the sequelae and the costs of these disorders. That requires adequate access to healthcare professionals, but also organizational efficiency using evidence and cost-effective-based diagnostic and therapeutic algorithms.

The imaging modalities available for the diagnosis of MSK disorders are multiple and both government and institutions have constantly supported a rigid step algorithm with the initial use of cheaper techniques (e.g., radiography), saving advanced modalities (e.g., CT and MRI) for the later stages. We believe that the choice of the imaging modality should be more tailored to each pathology and value-based, replacing the former cost-based, step algorithm. The knowledge of the values and limitations of the different imaging modalities should warrant the radiologist a central role in applying this change of management.

## 2 Choosing the Most Cost-Effective Technique: When and How

The inappropriate use of imaging exams regards its use against the recommendation of guidelines. It has been reported several times with the use of CT, for which increased costs are added to unnecessary radiation exposure. Griffith et al. (2014) evaluated the use of cervical spine CT in the emergency department after blunt trauma. Of the 1524 exams with negative findings, 364 (corresponding to 23.4%) were requested without following the guidelines. Some causes proposed by the authors for these requests were lack of knowledge or awareness/failure to remember the guidelines, lack of trust in them, difficulty in their interpretation/application, and clinical decision based on patient/scenario-specific factors.

The Ottawa ankle rules have also been developed to assist the selection of patients that should undergo radiography after trauma and which have negligible risk and therefore should have no imaging exams. The application of this guideline can help reduce the number of radiographs by 30% (Stiel et al. 1993).

Other factors linked to the rising costs in imaging departments are the heavy dependence of many MSK disorders' diagnostic criteria on MRI. Nevertheless, US is a cheaper modality, with superior space resolution, ability to better correlate imaging findings with patient symptoms, or capacity to perform dynamic studies. It has no contraindications and much of the times shows patient preference to MRI. US might in fact be more suited than MRI for some clinical indications (Klauser et al. 2012). Nevertheless, in 2005 Medicare MRI exams were nine times more frequent than US (Parker et al. 2008). Several reasons may explain the preference for MRI, namely the long learning curves or greater operator dependence of US, ability to reread the images, or the greater financial revenue of MRI (fee-for-service model). Also, the referring physicians might also find MRI images more standardized and easier to read, most of the times leading to a diagnosis without the use of other modalities.

Replacing US for MRI, when appropriate, could have a tremendous economic impact with cost-savings in the USA estimated to be around $736 million per year by 2020 (Parker et al. 2008). Therefore, MSK radiologists should master this technique worldwide, know its indications and limitations, and have a central role in its appropriate use. Referring physicians' habits or personal preference should be replaced by cost-efficient imaging guidelines directed to each clinical situation. Over the next paragraph we will present some daily cases in which the appropriate and cost-effective imaging approaches are discussed.

## 3 Case Scenario Approach

### 3.1 Case 1: Rotator Cuff Disease

35-Year-old male is seen by the orthopedic surgeon for complaints of shoulder pain. He reported sporadic sports practice and there was no history of trauma. Both clinical history and physical examination were consistent with rotator cuff pathology and the physician wanted to exclude a rotator cuff tear. Which imaging modalities should be used?

#### 3.1.1 Role of Imaging

Rotator cuff tears are the most common nontraumatic upper limb cause of disability in people over 50 years (Oliva et al. 2014) and the third most common cause of musculoskeletal consultation in primary care (Dinnes et al. 2003). Radiography is usually the first-line modality to be used in many institutions, usually followed by US or MRI, depending on the patient and local expertise.

#### 3.1.2 Rationale: A Value-Based Approach

Nazarian et al. (2013) provided an imaging algorithm for evaluating suspected rotator cuff disease after a multidisciplinary experts' consensus (including a healthcare economist). According to them, although radiography may be useful in all age groups, it is of low yield in patients younger than 40 years with no history of trauma. US should be the first modality to be used, considering its nearly equivalent accuracy to MR for complete and partial-thickness tears (Jesus et al. 2009), lower cost, greater acceptance, and no contraindications. They created an algorithm for the appropriate use of imaging techniques in shoulder pathologies. This is in accordance with

the European Society of Musculoskeletal Radiology (ESSR) Delphi-based consensus (Klauser et al. 2012), which also proposes US as the first-line modality in the diagnosis of bursitis, bicipital long-head rupture, or dislocation and septic arthritis. The workup might be completed with US and allow for appropriate treatment in many circumstances.

MRI might be used in the surgical cases, especially if there is retraction of the torn tendon medially to the acromion or in cases in which the US does not explain the patient symptoms. MR arthrography has shown greater accuracy in comparison to US and plain MRI for rotator cuff tears (Jesus et al. 2009), although its greater invasiveness should also be balanced in each case. It is the most appropriate examination in patients with shoulder instability, providing a more detailed assessment of the labrum and capsule-ligamentous structures.

The panel of experts involved in this algorithm (Nazarian et al. 2013) also highlighted the importance of an adequate clinical examination and consideration of local expertise in the choice of the imaging modality. The same factors, along with the respective availability of US and MRI, have also been highlighted in the Italian Society of Muscles, Ligaments and Tendons (I.S.Mu.L.T.) guidelines for rotator cuff pathology for the choice of the appropriate imaging technique to be used (Oliva et al. 2015).

---

**Key Points**

**Radiographs:** Are of low yield and can be avoided in patients up to 40 years old with suspected rotator cuff pathology and no history of trauma.

**US:** Has been proposed as the first-line modality in most uncomplicated cases.

**MRI:** Should be used in the surgical cases, mainly if there is retraction of the torn tendon medially to the acromion, or in cases in which US does not explain patient symptoms. MR arthrography provides greater accuracy in patients with joint instability.

## 3.2 Case 2: Scaphoid Fracture

Young adult female who reported a fall on the outstretched hand presented to the emergency department with wrist pain and tenderness on the anatomic snuffbox. The radiographs in two planes didn't reveal any traumatic lesions, although the orthopedic surgeon still suspected a scaphoid fracture based on the physical examination. What should be the best procedure?

### 3.2.1 Role of Imaging

Scaphoid fractures are common and represent 75% of all carpal bone fractures (Hauger et al. 2002). The incidence of occult fractures (with initial negative radiographs) is around 9% (Hauger et al. 2002). They may have a high morbidity if the diagnosis or appropriate treatment is delayed (nonunion, osteonecrosis, and osteoarthritis). Therefore, in order to reduce the risk of complications, conventional management usually involves a temporary (10–14 days) wrist cast followed by clinical and radiographic reassessment. Immobilization might be prolonged if the clinical suspicion persists, even when the radiographs remain negative for fracture.

### 3.2.2 Rationale: A Value-Based Approach

If the goal of this conventional strategy used in many institutions is to decrease the rate of complications and displacement of such fractures, it comes with the expense of long-period immobilization of many patients without fracture, with considerable reduced quality of life, work limitation, and healthcare costs associated with a close follow-up and overtreatment of patients without significant lesions. It should be mentioned that the positive predictive value of physical examination is as low as 21% (Dorsay et al. 2001). MRI is considered the most accurate imaging modality to identify occult early scaphoid fractures (Kusano et al. 2002). Nevertheless, its higher cost prevents its routine use in these patients. Patel et al. (2013) showed in a prospective study that the early use of MRI is marginally cost saving (£28.74 corresponding to 5.4% of the cost per patient) compared with the conventional treatment, justified by fewer outpatient appointments and follow-up radiographs. This approach was also associated with better pain and satisfaction scores. Similar economic savings were also reported in a retrospective study with 224 patients with an early MRI approach leading to savings of 92€ per patient (Moller et al. 2004). It should be stated that in addition to the social benefits of this early-MRI approach, the financial savings could greatly increase, depending on the cost per exam. A cost-effective analysis of this advanced imaging approach also concluded than even when combining the highest cost for advanced imaging and lowest costs for empiric immobilization and follow-up radiography, advanced imaging, particularly MRI, is still more cost effective (Karl et al. 2015).

Hauger et al. (2002) conducted a prospective study that showed sensitivity of 100% and a specificity of 98% of US to diagnose waist scaphoid fractures, using cortical disruption as the criterion. The great accuracy (sensitivity of 77.8–100% and specificity from 71.4 to 100%) of US in detecting occult waist scaphoid fractures was also shown in a recent review of the literature (Kwee and Kwee 2018), proving this technique to be cost effective when CT or MRI were not readily available.

> **Key Points**
>
> **Occult scaphoid fractures:** Their prevalence and its high rate of complications justify a great concern with the clinical impact of missed fractures.
>
> **MRI:** Several studies have shown cost-effectiveness in the use of advanced imaging techniques, particularly MRI, over the conventional strategy (immobilization followed by short-term clinical and radiographic follow-up).
>
> **US:** Might also be used in the evaluation of these patients, when MRI or CT is unavailable, with cortical disruption showing high accuracy for its diagnosis.

## 3.3 Case 3: Traumatic Hip Pain—Suspected Fracture

72-Year-old female presents to the emergency department with unilateral traumatic hip pain. There is no history of previous surgeries and she is otherwise healthy. The radiographs were negative, but the physician was still suspicious of femoral fracture. What is the appropriate next step to be taken?

### 3.3.1 Role of Imaging

Radiographs provide a sensitivity and specificity of around 90% and 98%, respectively, for femoral neck fractures (Cannon et al. 2009), so an occult fracture (with negative radiographs) remains a possibility. Moreover, these fractures are associated with increased morbidity, with great impact on autonomy and ability to perform daily activities. Also, a delay in surgery over 48 h is associated with a double increase in mortality at 1 year (Zuckerman et al. 1995). A common practice is to study these patients with CT to rule out occult fractures.

### 3.3.2 Rationale: A Value-Based Approach

Yun et al. (2016) compared the cost-effectiveness of four strategies in the diagnosis of occult hip fractures: discharging the patient if the radiographs were negative, only CT, only MRI, and MRI if CT was negative. In their analysis, obtaining an MRI was a better option than CT or discharging the patient. Initial CT followed by MRI if negative CT was a more expensive and less effective strategy. Even for facilities in urban areas, in which the cost of interfacility transportation is low, transferring the patient to an MRI-capable facility was more efficient than obtaining CT. In the NICE clinical guidelines for hip fractures (NICE 2018), it is also highlighted that MRI should be offered in suspected occult fractures and CT should be reserved for cases in which MRI is contraindicated or unavailable within 24 h.

**Key Points**
**Appropriateness of request:** Despite the high sensitivity of radiographs for hip fracture (90%), advanced imaging techniques should be done if an occult hip fracture is suspected.

**MRI:** It is the most cost-efficient modality in this regard. Even in an institution without MRI, transferring the patient to an MRI-capable facility might be the most cost-efficient strategy.

## 3.4 Case 4: Traumatic Knee Pain

A middle-aged male came to the emergency room complaining of knee pain after a trauma 2 days ago during a football match. He mentioned occasional sports practice and no previous surgeries. Knee radiographs were normal. What would be the most cost-efficient management option?

### 3.4.1 Role of Imaging

The practice in most hospitals in such a case would be to discharge the patient after a negative radiograph, eventually with a short-term consultation with his/her general practitioner. MRI is an established tool in the evaluation of acute knee trauma, providing an accurate diagnosis that allows to choose the optimal surgical or nonsurgical treatment. Nevertheless, considering its high cost and limited availability, it is usually not performed in the acute phase.

### 3.4.2 Rationale: A Value-Based Approach

Oei et al. (2009) developed a prospective study to assess the cost-effectiveness of a short protocol (6-min acquisition time) using low-field MRI in 208 patients with knee injury. They evaluated three strategies for management—radiography only, radiography plus MRI in all patients, and radiography followed by MRI only if radiographs were negative. They reduced image quality but showed equivalent diagnostic performances for most traumatic knee abnormalities with the advantage of lower cost and faster examinations. Total costs were lower in patients with MRI following a negative radiograph and higher in patients followed with radiography only, owing to lower productivity with the latter strategy. Other parameters, such as 6-week quality of life, time to diagnosis, or time to convalescence, were also better in the groups having an MRI. Moreover, the long time until some patients have a final diagnosis might lead to some physicians requesting a knee US for these patients, owing to its lower cost and higher accessibility. The use of this technique should be considered only in specific clinical scenarios and always following an accurate physical examination. In fact, the Delphi-based consensus on MSK ultrasound highlights that this modality should not be used if anterior/posterior cruciate ligaments or meniscal tears are suspected (Klauser et al. 2012).

**Key Points**
**Radiographs:** Have low sensitivity for displaying soft-tissue lesions associated with acute knee trauma.

**MRI:** The use of MRI with shorter protocols could allow cost savings compared to imaging strategies based on radiographs only. Short-term quality of life, time to diagnosis, and time to convalescence are also better in the former strategy.

**US:** Its use in knee trauma should be well judged clinically and its lack of accuracy for cruciate ligament and meniscal tear detection has to be considered.

# 4    Conclusion: Value-Based MSK Radiology

With the worldwide exponential growth in the use of ultrasound, among radiologists, non-radiologists, physicians, and other healthcare practitioners, new issues arise. Building expertise for MSK ultrasound is challenging, long-lasting, and becoming more heterogenous in this global demand for its use. Radiologists are usually taught in their residency by more experienced specialists or during postgraduate fellowships. For other physicians and other healthcare practitioners, there is a wide range of courses offered by different stakeholders.

In all cases, MSK ultrasound should be performed in a standard technique, with image documentation and a written report to assure adequate quality (Bureau and Ziegler 2016). Training or experience does not guarantee quality, so certification and accreditation should be mandatory, especially considering the great heterogeneity in formation and practice. Knowledge and competence should be important parameters when deciding who should perform imaging. Moreover, since many non-radiologists perform imaging in self-referred patients, the need for following appropriate guidelines gains relevance.

Despite its accessibility, lack of ionizing radiation, and lower cost of US compared to advanced imaging techniques, the medical, social, and economic consequences of its inappropriate use could be tremendous and remain to be well established. Inappropriate use of US might lead to duplication of exams, increased patient anxiety associated with false positives, or unrelevant clinical imaging findings. On the other hand, it can also lead to delay in the correct diagnosis in cases of false negatives so the questions of who and when should be addressed in considering MSK imaging.

The relevance of the referring physician's clinical skills cannot be overemphasized. The access to highly advanced imaging studies, even done with competent and experienced radiologists, does not assure appropriate patient management per se. Imaging findings should be precisely assessed to guarantee that they are clinically relevant and deserve treatment, but also to assure that patient symptoms can be fully explained by these imaging findings and there is no need to search for a synchronous disease.

## Key Points

- MSK ultrasound is highly valuable and its use is exponentially increasing worldwide, due to wide accessibility, lack of ionizing radiation, and lower cost. Certification and accreditation should be mandatory in order to provide appropriate quality.
- Potential high costs associated with false-positive or false-negative findings warrant the appropriate use of US performed by experienced and competent professionals.
- The use of MRI with shorter protocols has been considered, in many case scenarios, more cost effective than the conventional approach that only includes radiographs.
- Clinical correlation of all imaging findings is at least as important as a correct imaging diagnosis for patient management.

# References

Bureau NJ, Ziegler D (2016) Economics of musculoskeletal ultrasound. Curr Radiol Rep 4:44

Cannon J, Silvestri S, Munro M (2009) Imaging choices in occult hip fracture. J Emerg Med 37:144–152

Dinnes J, Loveman E, McIntyre L et al (2003) The effectiveness of diagnostic tests for the assessment of shoulder pain due to soft tissue disorders: a systematic review. Health Technol Assess 7(29):1–166

Dorsay TA, Major NM, Helms CA (2001) Cost-effectiveness of immediate MR imaging versus traditional follow-up for revealing radiographically occult scaphoid fractures. AJR Am J Roentgenol 177:1257–1263

Griffith B, Brown ML, Jain R (2014) Improving imaging utilization through practice quality improvement (maintenance of certification part IV): a review of requirements and approach to implementation. AJR Am J Roentgenol 202:797–802

Hauger BO, Moinard M et al (2002) Occult fractures of the waist of the scaphoid: early diagnosis by high-spatial-resolution sonography. AJR Am J Roentgenol 178:1239–1245

Jesus JO, Parker L, Frangos AJ et al (2009) Accuracy of MRI, MR arthrography, and ultrasound in the diagnosis of rotator cuff tears: a meta-analysis. AJR Am J Roentgenol 192(6):1701–1707

Karl JW, Swart E, Strauch RJ (2015) Diagnosis of occult scaphoid fractures: a cost-effectiveness analysis. J Bone Joint Surg Am 97:1860–1868

Klauser AS, Tagliafico A, Allen GM et al (2012) Clinical indications for musculoskeletal ultrasound: a Delphi-based consensus paper of the European society of musculoskeletal radiology. Eur Radiol 22:1140–1148

Kusano N, Churei Y, Shiraishi E et al (2002) Diagnosis of occult carpal scaphoid fracture: a comparison of magnetic resonance imaging and computed tomography techniques. Tech Hand Up Extrem Surg 6:119–123

Kwee RM, Kwee TC (2018) Ultrasound for diagnosing radiographically occult scaphoid fracture. Skelet Radiol 47(9):1205–1212

Moller JM, Larsen L, Bovin J et al (2004) MRI diagnosis of fracture of the scaphoid bone: impact of a new practice where the images are read by radiographers. Acad Radiol 11:724–728

Nazarian LN, Jacobson JA, Benson CB et al (2013) Imaging algorithms for evaluating suspected rotator cuff disease: society of radiologists in ultrasound consensus conference statement. Radiology 267:589–595

NICE (2018). https://www.nice.org.uk/guidance/cg124. Accessed 19 Oct 2018

Oei EH, Nikken JJ, Ginai AZ et al (2009) Costs and effectiveness of a brief MRI examination of patients with acute knee injury. Eur Radiol 19:409–418

Oliva F, Osti L, Padulo J et al (2014) Epidemiology of the rotator cuff tears: a new incidence related to thyroid disease. Muscle Ligaments Tendons J 4(3):309–314

Oliva F, Piccirilli E, Bossa M et al (2015) I.S.Mu.L.T. – rotator cuff tears guidelines. Muscles Ligaments Tendons J 5(4):227–263

Parker L, Nazarian L, Carrino JA et al (2008) Musculoskeletal imaging: medicare use, costs, and potential for cost substitution. J Am Coll Radiol 5:182–188

Patel NK, Davies N, Mirza Z et al (2013) Cost and clinical effectiveness of MRI in occult scaphoid fractures: a randomised controlled trial. Emerg Med J 30:202–207

Sharpe RE, Nazarian LN, Parker L et al (2012) Dramatically increased musculoskeletal ultrasound utilization from 2000 to 2009, especially by podiatrists in private offices. J Am Coll Radiol 9(2):141–146

Stiel IG, Greenberg GH, McKnight GH et al (1993) Decision rules for the use of radiography in acute ankle injuries: refinement and prospective validation. JAMA 269:1127–1132

Widanarko B, Legg S, Stevenson M et al (2012) Prevalence and work-related risk factors for reduced activities and absenteeism due to low back symptoms. Appl Ergon 43(4):727–737

Woolf AD (2000) The bone and joint decade 2000–2010. Ann Rheum Dis 59:81–82

Woolf AD, Plefger B (2003) Burden of major musculoskeletal conditions. Bull World Health Organ 81(9):646–656

Yun BJ, Hunink MG, Prabhakar AM et al (2016) Diagnostic imaging strategies for occult hip fractures: a decision and cost–effectiveness analysis. Acad Emerg Med 23:1161–1169

Zuckerman JD, Skovron ML, Koval KJ et al (1995) Postoperative complications and mortality associated with operative delay in older patients who have a fracture of the hip. J Bone Joint Surg Am 77:1551–1556

# Value-Based Radiology in Breast Imaging

Inês Leite and Elisa Melo Abreu

## Contents

I. Leite (✉)
Radiology Department, Santa Maria Hospital,
Lisbon, Portugal
e-mail: inex.leite@gmail.com

E. M. Abreu
Radiology Department, Porto University Hospital
Centre, Porto, Portugal

### Abstract

In this chapter, five common case presentations of everyday situations in the field of Breast Imaging are discussed.

We reinforce the importance of following best practice diagnostic guidelines in common issues, such as breast implant complications, assessment of nipple discharge, and the evaluation of the male symptomatic breast. Indeed, these guidelines are not always followed consistently in clinical practice which, in turn, has a direct negative effect on medical resource allocation decisions, contributing to expensive and ineffective procedures, with no additional benefit on healthcare outcomes.

We also highlight the role of MRI in the diagnosis and management of breast cancer. This technique combines excellent soft tissue contrast and detailed tumor angiogenesis information which contributes to its success in early cancer detection and in the assessment of treatment response after chemotherapy. Recently, it has also become clear that MRI is superior to mammography on ductal carcinoma in situ diagnosis (discussed in the last case scenario).

Finally, we hope that this overview is a useful tool not only for radiologists, including those not familiar with breast imaging, but also for the other members of the multidisciplinary teams composing breast units as well as general practitioners and other physicians that commonly refer symptomatic patients and seek a specialist opinion.

Med Radiol Diagn Imaging (2019)
https://doi.org/10.1007/174_2019_213, © Springer Nature Switzerland AG
Published Online: 25 July 2019

**Table 1** Five case scenarios and key points recommendations for imaging assessment

| Case | Issue | Key points |
|------|-------|-----------|
| Case 1 | Breast implant complications | • Asymptomatic women with silicone implants and women with saline implants (either symptomatic or asymptomatic): imaging is not recommended<br>• Symptomatic women with silicone implants: imaging assessment is mandatory |
| Case 2 | Symptomatic male breast enlargement | • Men presenting with symmetrical and typical clinical features of gynecomastia or pseudogynecomastia: imaging is not recommended<br>• Men presenting with asymmetrical and indeterminate breast abnormalities: imaging assessment is mandatory |
| Case 3 | Nipple discharge | • Women presenting with physiologic nipple discharge: imaging is not recommended<br>• Women presenting with pathological nipple discharge: imaging assessment is mandatory |
| Case 4 | Breast cancer in neoadjuvant setting | • Women with breast cancer proposed for neoadjuvant chemotherapy in order to perform a conserving breast surgery: mandatory tumor location and imaging assessment of tumor response<br>• Women with a resectable breast cancer proposed for neoadjuvant chemotherapy, in whom mastectomy is the expected surgical option (multicentric tumor, adjuvant radiotherapy contraindication, other cause): tumor location is not recommended; imaging assessment of tumor response is necessary |
| Case 5 | Ductal carcinoma in situ (DCIS) | • Women with suspicious mammographic microcalcifications: vacuum-assisted biopsy (VAB) mandatory; additional MR imaging assessment recommended |

# 1 Introduction

Five key case scenarios are summarized in Table 1, with the purpose of providing the best current evidence-based knowledge for a correct diagnostic pathway, while avoiding inappropriate or redundant imaging.

# 2 Case 1: Breast Implant Complications

A 45-year-old patient presents to our department complaining of left-sided breast pain. She had previous history of breast augmentation surgery with subpectoral silicone implants placement. There was a family history of breast cancer.

## 2.1 Role of Imaging: A Value-Based Approach

Decision-making about breast implant imaging assessment is based on the clinical history and the type of surgical procedure. Regarding clinical history, one of the starting points is that

imaging should be reserved for symptomatic patients. There is weak evidence supporting the benefits of generalized implant screening as these women should follow the existing breast cancer screening program instead. Major complications are usually clinically evident and, in this setting, additional information is mandatory (Lourenco et al. 2018).

Firstly, the temporal relation between symptom onset and surgery must be assessed, as complications vary between the early and late postoperative period (Hillard et al. 2017; Yang and Muradali 2011). Early complications include infection and hematoma. Meanwhile, late major complications include capsular contracture and implant rupture. Capsular contracture usually occurs during the first postoperative months (Yang and Muradali 2011). The risk of implant rupture increases with age, particularly 6–8 years after surgery (Hillard et al. 2017; Yang and Muradali 2011). Silicone implant ruptures can either be intracapsular or extracapsular, with the former comprising more than 80% of the cases (Yang and Muradali 2011). Breast implant-associated anaplastic large-cell lymphoma is a rare and recently recognized entity, also occurring as a delayed complication (De Boer et al. 2018; Juanpere et al. 2011). A recently diagnosed peri-implant effusion after the first year of surgery is suspicious and warrants fluid aspiration to confirm the diagnosis (Green et al. 2018).

Secondly, it is also important to know the purpose of breast implant surgery. The majority of cases are due to cosmetic reasons, but congenital malformations correction and reconstruction after mastectomy are other frequent indications for this procedure. The knowledge about congenital abnormalities might reduce false positives related to implant malpositioning. As for oncoplastic surgery, one should be aware of the higher risk of breast cancer and the lower detection rate of mammography, even when implant-displaced views, also called Ecklund views, are included in the protocol (Juanpere et al. 2011).

Regarding surgical technique, the radiologist should be aware of the type of implant placement (subpectoral, subglandular, or dual plane) and the type of implant itself. The most commonly seen implant type have a single lumen (either silicone or saline filled), but double lumen or reversed double lumen prosthesis may also be encountered (Juanpere et al. 2011; Green et al. 2018). Imaging is usually not indicated to assess saline implant complications, since its diagnosis should be made mostly on clinical grounds. Subsequent implant collapse and saline reabsorption occurs in cases of rupture (Lourenco et al. 2018).

In opposite, imaging is required if silicone implants complications are suspected (Lourenco et al. 2018; Seiler et al. 2017). While capsular contracture (the most common complication) is more easily diagnosed with clinical examination, most patients with implant rupture are asymptomatic (Juanpere et al. 2011; Green et al. 2018). In addition, clinical evaluation is unreliable in silicone implant rupture, and more than 50% of cases will be missed without imaging (Lourenco et al. 2018; Juanpere et al. 2011). The initial evaluation protocol for these patients should include mammography (Fig. 1) and ultrasound in patients older than 40 years or ultrasound alone in younger patients (particularly before 30 years).

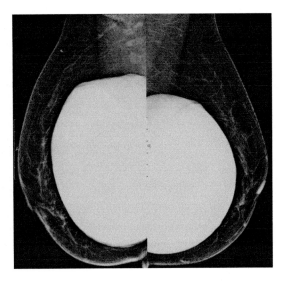

**Fig. 1** Mediolateral mammograms demonstrating no significant breast abnormalities regarding both silicone implants

Mammography and digital breast tomosynthesis (DBT) are not helpful in the diagnosis of intracapsular ruptures, but they often identify silicone outside the implant contour in the context of extracapsular ruptures (Lourenco et al. 2018; Seiler et al. 2017). Ultrasound has a high negative predictive value for implant rupture, with the most reliable sign being an anechoic appearance (Seiler et al. 2017). A true rupture is also usually confirmed whenever an implant rupture is suspected on ultrasound (Evans et al. 2018). The most reliable ultrasound signs for intracapsular and extracapsular ruptures are "the stepladder sign" (Fig. 2) and "the snowstorm" appearance of free silicone within either the breast gland or axillary lymph nodes, respectively (Yang and Muradali 2011; Juanpere et al. 2011; Seiler et al. 2017). Ultrasound-guided procedures such as biopsy and preoperative localization can be safely performed in women with breast implants (Evans et al. 2018).

Non-contrast-enhanced MRI is considered the most accurate technique and the modality of choice for implant integrity evaluation, with sensitivity and specificity above 90% in this setting (Hillard et al. 2017; Juanpere et al. 2011; Seiler et al. 2017). This technique is particularly helpful for intracapsular rupture diagnosis, which can be

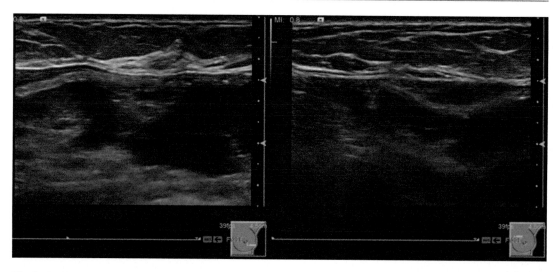

**Fig. 2** Breast ultrasound depicting multiple and discontinuous folds within the lumen of the left implant. This so-called "stepladder sign" is highly suggestive of intracapsular rupture

hard to diagnose with ultrasound and is usually clinically silent. In fact, some studies report sensitivity and specificity rates for ultrasound diagnosis of intracapsular ruptures as low as 30% and 77%, respectively (Lourenco et al. 2018; Evans et al. 2018; Scaranelo et al. 2004). The MRI hallmark sign of intracapsular rupture is the "linguini sign" (Fig. 3), which is characterized by the presence of curvilinear hypointense lines within the silicone gel (Yang and Muradali 2011; Juanpere et al. 2011; Seiler et al. 2017).

Breast MRI also accurately allows the differentiation of the type of implant rupture and provides a good assessment of the extent of granulomas and silicone leakage (namely to lymph nodes) related to extracapsular rupture (Lourenco et al. 2018; Juanpere et al. 2011). Dynamic contrast-enhanced MRI is recommended for high-risk women and for patients with history of oncoplastic reconstructive surgery, as to provide a better evaluation of breast parenchyma and increase cancer detection rates (Hillard et al. 2017; Juanpere et al. 2011; Seiler et al. 2017). Despite this, MRI should be reserved for the doubtful cases of implant integrity after conventional imaging and for the evaluation of silicone leakage extent in extracapsular rupture,

due to its elevated costs and limited availability (Juanpere et al. 2011; Seiler et al. 2017). Finally, comparison with prior tests is mandatory in women who had had prior silicone implant rupture to differentiate between leftover silicone and rupture of the new implant (Lourenco et al. 2018; Seiler et al. 2017).

## 2.2   Rationale

In this case scenario we start the evaluation with both mammography and ultrasound, given the patient's age and the absence of recent breast imaging studies. Mammography (Fig. 1) showed no significant abnormalities within the prosthesis, as is usually the case in intracapsular implant ruptures. Instead, the diagnosis was strongly suspected on ultrasound, which revealed multiple and discontinuous folds inside the lumen, the so-called "stepladder sign" (Fig. 2). The analogous "linguine sign" on MRI confirmed the intracapsular rupture (Fig. 3). Despite the absence of suspicious findings in the breast parenchyma, the MRI protocol included gadolinium-based contrast media injection, given the positive family history and the presence of dense breasts.

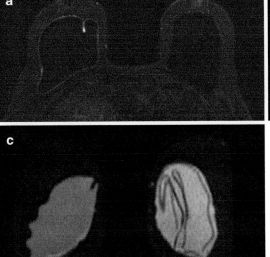

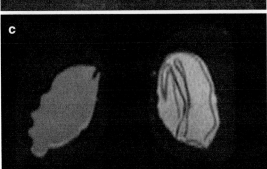

**Fig. 3** Breast MRI: (**a**) T2 weighted imaging (T2-WI) with fat saturation; (**b**, **c**) Silicone-only images [with both *short tau inversion recovery* (STIR) and *spectral* *attenuated inversion recovery* (SPAIR) pulses] confirming left intracapsular breast implant rupture—linguine sign. A radial fold is depicted in the intact right implant

**Key Points**
- Imaging is not routinely recommended for asymptomatic women with silicone implants and for women with saline implants (either symptomatic or asymptomatic).
- Symptomatic silicone implant complications require further imaging assessment.
- Both mammography and ultrasound are recommended as the initial exam in patients older than 40 years. Younger patients should be initially evaluated with ultrasound only.
- While MRI is the most accurate imaging modality, it should be reserved for high-risk patients, in doubtful cases of implant integrity after conventional imaging, and for the evaluation of silicone leakage extent.

## 3 Case 2: Symptomatic Male Breast Enlargement

A 41-year-old man was referred to our department with complaints of left-sided breast pain and tenderness. He had a previous medical history remarkable for alcoholic chronic liver disease and had started taking diuretics (spironolactone) 2 months before symptom onset. There were no signs of skin ulceration and no nipple discharge or retraction on physical examination. The family history for breast and testicular cancer was negative.

### 3.1 Role of Imaging: A Value-Based Approach

Most cases of symptomatic male breast alterations such as palpable breast mass or enlargement are benign, but clinical evaluation is mandatory due to concerns of breast cancer. Gynecomastia and pseudogynecomastia are the most common causes of palpable masses, accounting for up to 80% of tertiary referrals in the United States (Niell et al. 2018; Nguyen et al. 2013; Thiruchelvam et al. 2016). These conditions have a general population prevalence estimated between 32% and 65% (Desforges and Braunstein 1993). On the contrary, male breast cancer has a rather low incidence, with an average lifetime risk calculated around 1/1000 and a median age at diagnosis of 63 years (Niell et al. 2018). Thus, generalized male breast cancer screening programs are not justifiable. Instead, only men treated with exogenous hormone therapy for more than 5 years and transgender male to female patients older than 50 years of age should be systematically screened due to the increased risk of breast cancer (Chesebro et al. 2018).

The first step on the evaluation of the symptomatic male breast is a detailed clinical history and physical examination (Thiruchelvam et al. 2016). An exhaustive investigation must be conducted to identify any possible causes of gynecomastia associated to testosterone-to-estrogen ratio imbalance, including systemic diseases, recent weight gain or loss, or as a side effect of exogenous hormone use or recreational drugs. Family history should also be obtained, particularly to identify BRCA-2 mutation carriers, since they have a significant higher lifetime risk for breast cancer. The physical examination is conveyed to differentiate between gynecomastia and pseudogynecomastia and to rule out any suspicious clinical features for breast cancer, including unusual asymmetries, eccentric nodules, nipple retraction or discharge and associated axillary lymphadenopathy (Thiruchelvam et al. 2016).

This initial clinical approach has been proved to be very cost-effective since it can obviate unnecessary imaging workup when clinical assessment is consistent with typical and bilateral gynecomastia or pseudogynecomastia (Niell et al. 2018). This approach is mandatory to optimize medical resources and help reduce the excessive number of male mammography which have had a two- to threefold increase during the last decade, when comparing to the total

number of mammograms (Iuanow et al. 2011). Meanwhile, controversy remains on whether any imaging is needed for adult patients referring typical but unilateral symptoms of these conditions (Niell et al. 2018). The efficacy of unilateral incidences compared to bilateral mammography (Fig. 4) in these patients has not yet been evaluated (Niell et al. 2018).

Breast imaging is warranted in patients with inconclusive or suspicious clinical features. The selection of the first imaging modality depends on patient's age (Niell et al. 2018). It is important to be aware that this takes into account the age distribution of both gynecomastia and breast cancer. While gynecomastia has a bimodal prevalence, with a first peak near puberty (90% of cases being transitory) and a second peak in the fifth and sixth decades, breast cancer has a peak incidence in the sixth decade and is extremely rare before fourth decade, comprising less than 1% of cases (Nguyen et al. 2013; Thiruchelvam et al. 2016).

According to ACR Appropriateness Criteria, patients younger than 25 years old should perform ultrasound first, considering the risk of radiation exposure and the low probability of breast cancer in this age group. In the few cases in which ultrasound is inconclusive or has

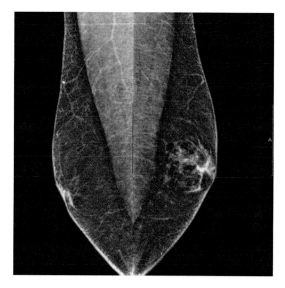

**Fig. 4** Mediolateral mammograms depicting asymmetrical gynecomastia of dendritic type (left predominant)

suspicious findings, mammography should then be performed (Niell et al. 2018).

Mammography or DBT are recommended as the first exam in patients older than 25 years since they have a high sensitivity, specificity, and negative predictive value for malignancy (above 90%) (Niell et al. 2018; Desforges and Braunstein 1993). The fact that these techniques have the potential to identify microcalcifications contributes to the better accuracy of breast cancer detection compared to ultrasound. There is weak evidence of the incremental benefit of DBT compared to mammography. Male breast cancer tends to manifest as peripheral or eccentric noncalcified masses or as noncontiguous foci of asymmetric density, most frequently sparing the subareolar region (Nguyen et al. 2013; Desforges and Braunstein 1993). However, it can also occur in association with calcifications and even round ones should be considered suspicious in male patients.

Studies have shown that targeted ultrasound has no additional value in patients with negative mammograms and in patients with typical gynecomastia or pseudogynecomastia at mammography. Indeed, false positive rates can be as high as 20%, leading to unnecessary biopsies and avoidable healthcare costs (Niell et al. 2018; Desforges and Braunstein 1993). There is also no benefit in further evaluation with mammography when characteristic imaging findings of gynecomastia are incidentally detected on CT scans and in the absence of suspicious clinical features (Niell et al. 2018). Currently, there are no clear guidelines on the use of breast MRI in the setting of suspected gynecomastia or during the evaluation of indeterminate palpable breast masses (Niell et al. 2018; Appelbaum et al. 1999).

In the presence of suspicious findings either at physical examination or at the initial imaging evaluation, both mammography or DBT and ultrasound should be conducted before biopsy (Niell et al. 2018; Desforges and Braunstein 1993). Ultrasound should include axillary evaluation, since 50% of men have nodal metastasis at the initial diagnosis of breast cancer (Nguyen et al. 2013). The literature suggests that breast cancer and gynecomastia usually coexist in approximately 50% of cases, though there is no clear evidence that gynecomastia increases cancer risk (Niell et al. 2018; Appelbaum et al. 1999). The clinical usefulness of breast MRI in male patients with breast cancer is still under debate (Niell et al. 2018; Shin et al. 2018).

## 3.2 Rationale

The rationale behind this case hinged on the fact that the patient's complaints were asymmetrical. Even though physical examination and previous medical history were very suggestive of gynecomastia, further imaging evaluation was conducted to confirm the diagnosis and exclude breast cancer beyond reasonable doubt. Mammography was the initial imaging modality of choice, due to the patient's age. Typical imaging findings of the dendritic type of gynecomastia were found (Fig. 4), characterized by the presence of a subareolar mass with radiating extensions into the subareolar fat. Breast ultrasound was deemed unnecessary given the unremarkable radiological findings.

**Key Points**

- Patients with symmetrical and tender breast enlargement consistent with gynecomastia or pseudogynecomastia do not need further imaging evaluation.
- For patients with indeterminate palpable masses the first imaging modality depends on the patient's age. Men older than 25 years should start their imaging evaluation with mammography, which has a high negative predictive value for breast cancer, avoiding additional ultrasound and biopsy when the exam is either negative or consistent with gynecomastia. In younger patients, ultrasound is recommended first.
- In the presence of suspicious findings, either at physical examination or at the initial imaging evaluation, both mammography and ultrasound are mandatory.

## 4    Case 3: Nipple Discharge

A 45-year-old woman complaining of left-sided bloody nipple discharge was referred to our department. The discharge was spontaneous and came out through a single pore. The physical examination was otherwise normal. There was no family history of breast cancer.

## 4.1    Role of Imaging: A Value-Based Approach

Nipple discharge is the third most common cause of breast imaging referral, after breast pain and palpable lumps, with an estimated incidence of 5–10% (Lippa et al. 2015).

The first step when evaluating nipple discharge is based on the clinical differentiation between physiological and pathological discharge which directs the need for further imaging evaluation (Lee et al. 2017). The assessment should be focused on nipple inspection and on the characteristics of the discharge (Paula and Campos 2017). Nonetheless, a general breast evaluation and a thorough clinical history (including age, hormone status, medical history and personal or family history of breast or ovarian cancer) is also mandatory.

Physiological discharge is typically bilateral, nonspontaneous, multiple pore, and milky or greenish in color. In the absence of other symptoms and with recent negative exams (within the last 6 months), further breast imaging is unnecessary, according to ACR Appropriateness Criteria (Lee et al. 2017). Hormonal changes, namely those related to pregnancy or breast-feeding, are the main causes of physiological discharge and are usually sorted out after a 2-year follow-up. Other causes of physiological discharge include various medications as well as breast disease such as galactophore ductal ectasia, fibrocystic disease, or periductal mastitis (Lippa et al. 2015; Lee et al. 2017).

On the other hand, pathological nipple discharge mandates imaging and is typically unilateral, spontaneous, single or pauci-pore and serous or hematic in color. It is associated with a higher risk of malignancy, particularly when it presents with palpable abnormalities (61.5% versus 6.1% when palpable abnormalities absent) (Lee et al. 2017; Cohen and Leung 2018). Papillomas (35–48%) and galactophore ductal ectasia (17–36%) are the most commonly found conditions (Cohen and Leung 2018). However, breast cancer, particularly DCIS, comprises 5–21% of the cases overall, with even higher incidences in males (23–57%) and women older than 60 years (32%) (Lippa et al. 2015; Lee et al. 2017; Cohen and Leung 2018).

Nipple smear cytology is of limited value, since false negative rates exceeds 50% for breast cancer detection (Lippa et al. 2015; Lee et al. 2017). Therefore, nipple smear cytology is no longer recommended in routine clinical practice.

Breast imaging usually correctly identifies and localizes the process responsible for pathologic nipple discharge and in most of the cases allows for a correct differentiation between benign and malignant or high-risk lesions. Thus, it plays a major role in healthcare cost reduction, minimizing the number of surgeries, limiting the extent of resection, and enabling minimally invasive procedures, such as percutaneous vacuum-assisted excision guided by imaging (Cohen and Leung 2018; Li et al. 2018; Patel et al. 2018; Panzironi et al. 2019). In fact, the latter procedure has a role in the resection of small intraductal papillary lesions with permanent cessation of nipple discharge reported to be as high as 90% (Lee et al. 2017).

A recently published study reported that radiologists do not consistently follow ACR Appropriateness Criteria regarding nipple discharge. This leads to a significant heterogeneity in the imaging modality workup and to unnecessary and avoidable medical costs (Patel et al. 2018). According to ACR Appropriateness Criteria, mammography (Fig. 5) or DBT should be the first imaging modalities in patients older than 39 years, though ultrasound is also usually performed. For women between 30 and 39 years

**Fig. 5** Mediolateral views showing bilateral dense breasts and nonspecific calcifications in the left subareolar region. A lymph node is also visible, located in the upper outer quadrant of the left breast

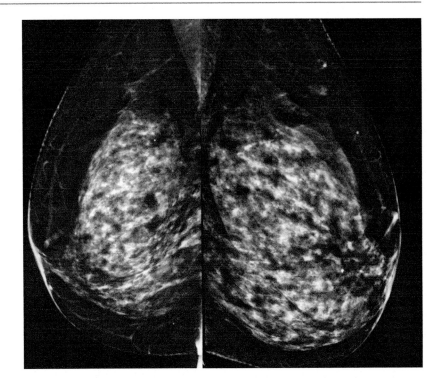

old, either mammogram or ultrasound are acceptable techniques. In women younger than 30 years, ultrasound is the modality of choice (Lee et al. 2017; Cohen and Leung 2018; Panzironi et al. 2019). The combined use of mammography or DBT and ultrasound is advocated whenever each of these techniques shows suspicious or indeterminate findings, regardless of age (Lee et al. 2017; Panzironi et al. 2019; Berger et al. 2017).

There is limited data on the usefulness of DBT compared to digital mammography (Lee et al. 2017). Women with unilateral symptoms should perform only unilateral mammograms to the affected breast once they had a recent four-view negative mammogram (Lee et al. 2017). Mammography has the potential to identify microcalcifications, which are typically associated to DCIS and are frequently morphologically distinct from the ones related to papillomas and plasmocytic mastitis, especially when they have

ductal, branching and segmental distributions. However, some papillomas have intralesional calcifications that can be suspicious at mammography and mimic DCIS. Furthermore, mammography has a low sensitivity (20–25%), particularly for the detection of retroareolar lesions and small noncalcified intraductal papillomas, even when magnified or localized spot compression views are performed (Lippa et al. 2015). Ultrasound with color Doppler assessment has a higher sensitivity (56–80%) compared to mammography in this setting, enabling better visualization of intraductal lesions (Lippa et al. 2015; Lee et al. 2017; Panzironi et al. 2019). However, this comes at the cost of reduced specificity when compared to mammography in differentiating between benign and malignant diseases (61–75%) (Lee et al. 2017). The utility of elastography remains under debate (Panzironi et al. 2019). One should take into account that isolated anechoic focal ductal dilatations (Fig. 6) also require further

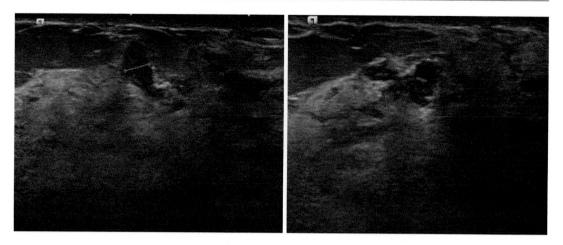

**Fig. 6** Breast ultrasound showing a hypoechoic intraluminal lesion arising from a single duct in the left breast

investigation, with papillomas and carcinomas being identified in 50% and 14% of cases, respectively (Lippa et al. 2015).

Contrast-Enhanced Breast MRI is now the gold standard modality when the initial standard imaging with mammography and ultrasound is negative or inconclusive, being an effective alternative to galactography and surgery, which have been traditional approaches in the past (Paula and Campos 2017; Cohen and Leung 2018; Li et al. 2018; Berger et al. 2017). Contrast-Enhanced Breast MRI is the technique with the highest sensitivity for breast cancer detection, ranging from 90% to 99%. It also allows bilateral breast imaging and correct visualization of the retroareolar and deeper posterior regions, thus enabling the detection of multifocal or multicentric disease and the identification of occult contralateral lesions (Cohen and Leung 2018; Panzironi et al. 2019; Berger et al. 2017). Nonetheless, some authors report low specificity (around 76%) and highlight the importance of performing a second-look ultrasound to help reduce the false positive rates and preclude excessive biopsies or surgeries (Paula and Campos 2017; Panzironi et al. 2019).

Breast MRI is reported to have higher sensitivity (88–95% versus 50–75%) and negative predictive value (98% versus 93%) for cancer detection when compared to galactography. The inability to detect multiple duct abnormalities as well as extraductal and posterior lesions is a clear drawback of galactography, with false negative rates estimated between 20% and 30% (Lee et al. 2017; Paula and Campos 2017; Panzironi et al. 2019; Berger et al. 2017). This technique also carries a considerable risk of complications (such as mastitis and ductal perforation) and is technically inadequate or incomplete in up to 20% of the cases (Panzironi et al. 2019). Although it has been gradually replaced by MRI, it is still valuable in some centers for preoperative topography in order to guide and optimize surgical planning. In fact, lesions with a distance from the nipple greater than 3 cm may not be resected, even with major duct excision, unless their exact location is spotted on imaging, either by MRI (Fig. 7) or galactography (Lee et al. 2017).

MRI is also crucial in deciding between conservative management and surgery, due to its high negative predictive value for cancer and high-risk lesions. If there are no suspicious findings on conventional imaging and MRI, then short-term surveillance (every 6 months for 2 years) is advised, avoiding unnecessary surgery (Paula and Campos 2017; Li et al. 2018; Panzironi et al. 2019). Recent studies report very few false negative cases of breast cancer when using breast MRI (4%), mostly comprising low grade DCIS or small invasive ductal carcinomas with overall favorable outcomes (Lippa et al. 2015; Li et al. 2018). Meanwhile, in the presence of diagnostic findings on MRI, excessive nipple discharge

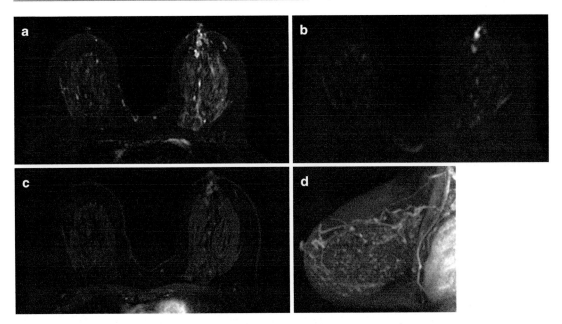

**Fig. 7** Breast MRI: (**a**) T2-WI with fat saturation; (**b**) diffusion-weighted image with $b = 800$; (**c**) early postcontrast image; (**d**) subtraction sagittal MIP. An elongated and hypervascularized lesion within a single duct in the subareolar region of the breast gland is clearly depicted. The lesion shows high signal intensity on both T2 weighted and diffusion imaging

and/or bothersome symptoms, surgery is recommended (Li et al. 2018; Panzironi et al. 2019).

## 4.2 Rationale

The rationale behind this case study approach was based on the worrisome features of nipple discharge, which mandated additional imaging. Both mammography and ultrasound were performed, given the patient's age and absence of prior breast imaging examinations in the last 6 months. Mammography revealed nonspecific subareolar microcalcifications (Fig. 5) and ultrasound revealed a hypoechoic lesion within a single central duct (Fig. 6), with a vascular stalk suspected on color Doppler (not shown). A percutaneous breast-guided biopsy was conducted and the result was consistent with a large solitary intraductal papilloma. Breast MRI (Fig. 7) was also performed to confirm the lesion extension and further exclude other pathological findings. The lesion was surgically resected once its dimensions exceeded 3 cm, precluding a percutaneous vacuum-assisted excision.

**Key Points**
- Breast imaging is not routinely recommended for the evaluation of physiologic nipple discharge.
- Imaging workup is required for all patients presenting with pathological nipple discharge. The selection of the correct modality depends on the patient's age.
- Mammography should be the first imaging modality for women older than 39 years, while women younger than 30 years should perform ultrasound first. Between 30 and 39 years of age, either ultrasound or mammography may be appropriate. The combined use of both techniques is indicated if suspicious or inconclusive findings are detected.
- When both mammography and ultrasound are negative, breast MRI should be performed to help guide the decision between conservative management and a surgical approach.

## 5    Case 4: Breast Cancer in Neoadjuvant Setting

A 62-year-old woman was referred to our department presenting with a painless lump in her left breast. There were no predisposing risk factors for breast cancer. A diagnostic bilateral mammogram was performed, revealing a highly suspicious nodule in the inner upper quadrant of her left breast. No axillary enlarged lymph nodes were found on complementary ultrasound. An ultrasound-guided core biopsy was made using an automated 14-gauge needle, and the pathological analysis revealed the diagnosis of invasive cancer with no special type, nuclear grade 3. Estrogen (ER), progesterone receptors (PR), and epidermal growth factor receptor 2 (HER2) were negative in all cells, and the Ki67 expression was about 70%. The patient underwent neoadjuvant chemotherapy, and the final analysis of the surgical specimen revealed a complete pathological response.

### 5.1    Role of Imaging: A Value-Based Approach

Decision-making on breast imaging in the neoadjuvant setting should be done according to the impact on the therapeutic strategy. It is important to perform an appropriate initial imaging locoregional staging in all patients with breast cancer.

Although the National Comprehensive Cancer Network (NCCN) guidelines recommend bilateral mammogram, ultrasound only as necessary and optional breast MR imaging with special consideration for mammography occult tumors, we not only emphasize that complementary ultrasound is crucial, particularly in evaluation of axillary lymph nodes, but also believe that breast MR imaging should be performed as well, since it is not possible to know if a breast cancer has additional mammographic occult DCIS, multifocal, multicentric or bilateral invasive components without performing this technique (National Comprehensive Cancer Network 2018). Multiple clinical trials show that MRI can detect occult disease in the ipsilateral breast in approximately 15% of patients, with ranges reported from 12% to 27% and disease in the contralateral breast in 4.3% to 5% of patients.

MRI determines disease extent more accurately than mammography and physical examination in many patients (American College of Radiology 2018).

On the other hand, there are no established clinical practice guidelines for how best to assess tumor response to neoadjuvant chemotherapy (Fowler et al. 2017). Scheel et al. analyzed the accuracy of preoperative measurements by clinical examination, mammography, and MR imaging for detecting pathologic complete response and association with final pathology size in women with ≥3 cm invasive breast cancer receiving neoadjuvant chemotherapy, and concluded that MR imaging showed the highest accuracy for detecting pathologic complete response, results that were not significantly influenced by tumor subtype or mammographic density (Scheel et al. 2018). Breast MRI may be useful before, during, and/or after chemotherapy to evaluate treatment response and the extent of residual disease prior to surgical treatment (American College of Radiology 2018).

Benefits of neoadjuvant chemotherapy include reducing tumor size before surgery and potentially convert a mastectomy to partial mastectomy or lumpectomy. As breast conservation in neoadjuvant setting still remains an important goal, we believe the assessment of tumor response should also include breast MRI. If combined with lesion bracketing that helps to translate the imaging information into the operating room, MR imaging for treatment planning is associated with a final positive margin rate that is overall low, and that does not differ for women with DCIS components versus women without DCIS components (Kuhl et al. 2017). In the event of complete response, localization tissue markers placed prior to neoadjuvant chemotherapy will indicate the location of the initial tumor (American College of Radiology 2018).

It is also important to understand the influence of tumor morphology and tumor phenotype in the accuracy of breast MRI, to understand when a complete response in this technique is effectively able to predict a pathological complete response. Several studies have shown that well-circumscribed solid lesions, which are HER2 positive, triple negative, or reveal high Ki67 index, demonstrate higher probability of concentric and complete response (versus partial and fragmented response in positive ER positive tumors), and better concordance between post-neoadjuvant chemotherapy tumor size on MR imaging and on surgical specimen (McGuire et al. 2011; Mukhtar et al. 2013). The placement of radiopaque markers for tumor location in patients undergoing neoadjuvant chemotherapy and breast conserving surgery should also be done according to tumor phenotype and expected pattern of response (Youn et al. 2015).

At the moment, the impact of tumor phenotype and complete MR imaging response on surgical treatment planning is to allow a more conserving breast surgery. Despite MR imaging promising data, it is not currently reliable enough to allow patients to avoid surgical resection after complete imaging response. Clinical trials are trying to understand if selected patients who present an imaging complete response after neoadjuvant chemotherapy can avoid surgical resection in the future (American College of Radiology 2018; Kuerer et al. 2018).

## 5.2 Rationale

In this case scenario we started the evaluation with both mammography (Fig. 8a, b) and ultrasound, followed by ultrasound-guided breast biopsy. The initial locoregional staging included breast MRI (Fig. 9), which confirmed a unifocal circumscribed solid lesion, without significant occult mammography components. Given the

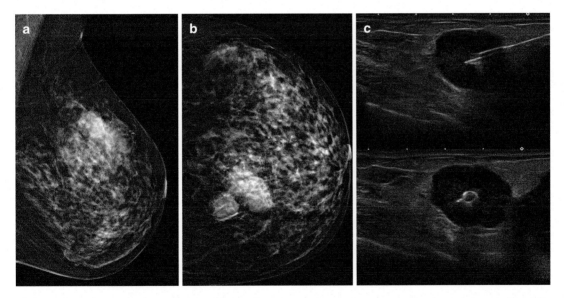

**Fig. 8** (a) Mediolateral oblique and (b) craniocaudal projections showing a heterogeneously dense left breast with a unifocal circumscribed solid lesion in the inner upper quadrant. (c) Since the patient was considered potentially eligible for breast conserving treatment, tumor location was performed under ultrasound guidance

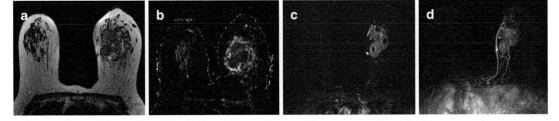

**Fig. 9** Pre-neoadjuvant chemotherapy breast MRI. (a) Axial T2-WI, (b) Apparent diffusion coefficient (ADC) map, (c) T1-WI with fat saturation (T1FS) subtraction image, and (d) Maximal Intensity Projection (MIP) image showing a highly suspicious hypointense unifocal solid lesion in the inner upper quadrant of the left breast, revealing restriction in diffusion sequence and heterogeneous enhancement in dynamic acquisition, with washout type of time-intensity kinetic curve

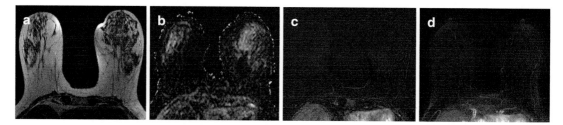

**Fig. 10** Post-neoadjuvant chemotherapy breast MRI. (**a**) Axial T2-WI, (**b**) ADC map, (**c**) T1FS subtraction image, and (**d**) MIP image showing a complete imaging response

triple negative tumor subtype and initial staging (T2N0), the patient was proposed for neoadjuvant chemotherapy. Since she was considered potentially eligible for breast conserving treatment, radiopaque markers for tumor location were placed under ultrasound guidance (Fig. 8c). After neoadjuvant chemotherapy, the patient revealed a MR imaging complete response (Fig. 10). As there is a high accuracy of MR imaging in these morphology and phenotype subtype tumor, a more conserving breast surgery was proposed. The final analysis of the surgical specimen confirmed the complete pathological response.

> **Key Points**
> - MR imaging is the most accurate method to analyze the tumor response.
> - High accuracy of MRI in estimating post-chemotherapy tumor response occurs on well-circumscribed solid lesions, triple negative and HER2+ subtypes. Particularly in this setting, MR imaging is a reliable method to assess the neoadjuvant chemotherapy use for downstaging patients to be eligible for breast conserving treatment.
> - Despite promising data, MRI is not yet reliable enough to allow patients to avoid surgical resection after complete imaging response. Clinical trials are trying to understand if selected patients can avoid breast surgery.
> - Tumor location in patients undergoing neoadjuvant chemotherapy and breast conserving surgery should be done according to tumor phenotype and expected pattern of response.

## 6    Case 5: Ductal Carcinoma In Situ

A 53-year-old woman was referred to our department presenting an abnormal right breast screening mammogram. She was asymptomatic, and there were no predisposing risk factors for breast cancer.

In the upper outer quadrant of her right breast, we found coarse heterogeneous microcalcifications with segmental distribution, suspicious for malignancy.

A stereotactic VAB was performed using a 7-gauge needle, and the pathological analysis revealed the diagnosis of DCIS of intermediate nuclear grade, with solid pattern and comedonecrosis, positive ER in 98% of the cells. The patient underwent breast conserving breast surgery, followed by adjuvant radio- and hormonotherapy.

### 6.1    Role of Imaging: A Value-Based Approach

Decision-making on breast imaging in suspicious microcalcifications and DCIS remains somewhat controversial. If VAB already proved its benefits when compared to core-needle biopsy of microcalcifications and is well established, the overdiagnosis versus overtreatment issue, and the diagnostic value of breast MRI still remain under intense debate.

Effectively, a recent meta-analysis compared the diagnostic performance of VAB and core needle biopsy for microcalcifications, endorsing the better diagnostic performance of VAB in DCIS underestimation rate and microcalcifications retrieval rate (Huang et al. 2018).

With the widespread adoption of population-based breast cancer screening, DCIS has come to represent 20–25% of all breast cancers. Currently, surgical treatment followed by radiotherapy as part of breast conserving treatment, and potentially additional adjuvant hormone therapy, aims preventing invasive breast cancer, although a significant proportion of DCIS lesions may never progress. This fact is responsible for overtreatment of DCIS which would never evolve to invasive carcinoma, and has motivated the beginning of clinical trials of active surveillance such as LORIS or LORD study, which aims to understand if it is possible sparing a selected group of DCIS from such unnecessary treatment (Francis et al. 2015; Elshof et al. 2015; Groen et al. 2017).

In order to allow an appropriate evaluation of the disease extension, including non-calcifying DCIS, breast MRI has emerged as an imaging biomarker of aggressiveness (potentially differentiating between low grade and high nuclear grade), which can stage and depict invasive foci better than mammography, if used in specialized breast centers, with optimized MRI protocols and interpreted by experienced breast radiologists.

Finally, recently it was shown that MRI might be used to accurately distinguish benign from malignant mammographic microcalcifications, helping to reduce unnecessary breast biopsies (Baltzer et al. 2018).

## 6.2 Rationale

In this case scenario we started the evaluation with mammography and additional magnified views (Fig. 11) to better depict microcalcifications morphology and distribution. As microcalcifications were considered suspicious for malignancy, a stereotaxic-guided breast VAB using a 7G needle was performed, and 12 samples were obtained with satisfactory retrieval of microcalcifications (Fig. 12). A small marker was placed in the breast biopsy site.

**Fig. 11** (a) Mediolateral oblique view of the right breast and (b) spot magnification view showing amorphous microcalcifications with segmental distribution, classified as BI-RADS 4B. (c) Radiograph of breast conserving surgical specimen

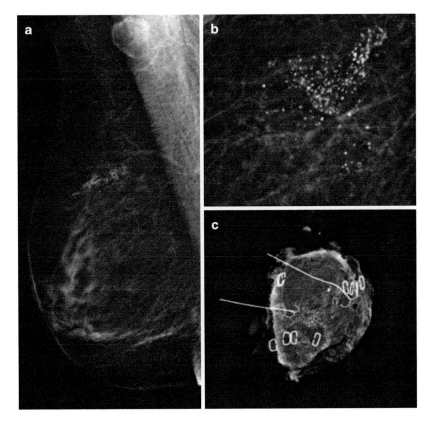

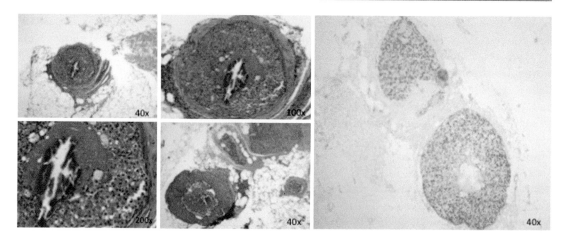

**Fig. 12** Pathologic findings at VAB revealed the diagnosis of DCIS of intermediate nuclear grade, with solid pattern and comedonecrosis, positive ER in 98% of cells

As there is a higher accuracy of MRI to evaluate the disease extension, it is recommended performing a MRI staging previously to the conserving therapy. As stated in the previous case scenario, if combined with nonsurgical biopsy methods (MR-guided vacuum biopsy), and with methods that help translate the imaging information into the operating room (MR-guided lesion bracketing), MRI for treatment planning is associated with an overall lower positive margin rate, even in cases of DCIS (Kuhl et al. 2017).

**Key Points**
- MRI is the most accurate method to analyze the disease extension, including noncalcified DCIS.
- VAB has better diagnostic performance in DCIS, when compared with core needle biopsy, revealing lower underestimation rate and higher microcalcifications retrieval rate.
- If combined with MR-guided vacuum biopsy and with lesion bracketing, MRI for treatment planning is associated with an overall lower positive margin rate.

## 7 Summary

The selected case scenarios illustrate and help to understand the importance of applying best practice diagnostic guidelines to common breast issues: breast implant complications, nipple discharge and symptomatic male breast evaluation, to enable optimal allocation of medical resources and healthcare outcomes. The contribution of MRI for the diagnosis and management of breast cancer is also highlighted in the last two cases. We hope that this chapter is valuable not only for radiologists, but also for other members of breast multidisciplinary teams and general practitioners.

## References

American College of Radiology (2018) ACR practice parameter for the performance of contrast-enhanced magnetic resonance imaging (MRI) of the breast (Resolution 34). Revised 2018. Accessed 25 Sept 2018

Appelbaum AH, Evans GF, Levy KR, Amirkhan RH, Schumpert TD (1999) Mammographic appearances of male breast disease. Radiographics 19(3): 559–568

Baltzer P et al (2018) Is breast MRI a helpful additional diagnostic test in suspicious mammographic microcalcifications? Magn Reson Imaging 46:70–74

Berger N, Luparia A, Di Leo G, Carbonaro LA, Trimboli RM, Ambrogi F, Sardanelli F (2017) Diagnostic performance of MRI versus galactography in women with pathologic nipple discharge: a systematic review and meta-analysis. AJR Am J Roentgenol 209(2):465–471

Chesebro AL, Rives AF, Shaffer K (2018) Male breast disease: what the radiologist needs to know. Curr Probl Diagn Radiol (in press), accepted manuscript. Available online 29 Jul. pii: S0363-0188(18)30061-6

Cohen E, Leung JWT (2018) Problem-solving MR imaging for equivocal imaging findings and indeterminate clinical symptoms of the breast. Magn Reson Imaging Clin N Am 26(2):221–233

De Boer M, van Leeuwen FE, Hauptmann M, Overbeek LIH, de Boer JP, Hijmering NJ, de Jong D (2018) Breast implants and the risk of anaplastic large-cell lymphoma in the breast. JAMA Oncol 4(3):335–341

Desforges JF, Braunstein GD (1993) Gynecomastia. New Engl J Med 328:490–495

Elshof EL et al (2015) Feasibility of a prospective, randomised, open-label, international multicentre, phase III, non-inferiority trial to assess the safety of active surveillance for low risk ductal carcinoma in situ—the LORD study. Eur J Cancer 51:1497–1510

Evans A, Trimboli RM, Athanasiou A, Balleyguier C, Baltzer PA, Bick U, Camps Herrero J, Clauser P, Colin C, Cornford E, Fallenberg EM, Fuchsjaeger MH, Gilbert FJ, Helbich TH, Kinkel K, Heywang-Köbrunner SH, Kuhl CK, Mann RM, Martincich L, Panizza P, Pediconi F, Pijnappel RM, Pinker K, Zackrisson S, Forrai G, Sardanelli F, European Society of Breast Imaging (EUSOBI), with language review by Europa Donna—The European Breast Cancer Coalition (2018) Breast ultrasound: recommendations for information to women and referring physicians by the European Society of Breast Imaging. Insights Imaging 9(4):449–461

Fowler AM, Mankoff DA, Bonnie NJ (2017) Imaging neoadjuvant therapy response in breast cancer. Radiology 285(2):358–375

Francis A et al (2015) LORIS trial: addressing overtreatment of ductal carcinoma in situ. Clin Oncol 27:6–8

Green LA, Karow JA, Toman JE, Lostumbo A, Xie K (2018) Review of breast augmentation and reconstruction for the radiologist with emphasis on MRI. Clin Imaging 47:101–117

Groen EJ et al (2017) Finding the balance between over- and under-treatment of ductal carcinoma in situ (DCIS). Breast 31:274–283

Hillard C, Fowler JD, Barta R, Cunningham B (2017) Silicone breast implant rupture: a review. Gland Surg 6(2):163–168

Huang XC et al (2018) A comparison of diagnostic performance of vacuum-assisted biopsy and core needle biopsy for breast microcalcification: a systematic review and meta-analysis. Ir J Med Sci 187(4):999–1008

Iuanow E, Kettler M, Slanetz PJ (2011) Spectrum of disease in the male breast. AJR Am J Roentgenol 196(3):247–259

Juanpere S, Perez E, Huc O, Motos N, Pont J, Pedraza S (2011) Imaging of breast implants—a pictorial review. Insights Imaging 2(6):653–670

Kuerer HM et al (2018) A clinical feasibility trial for identification of exceptional responders in whom breast cancer surgery can be eliminated following neoadjuvant systemic therapy. Ann Surg 267:946–951

Kuhl C, Strobel K, Bleling K, Wardelmann E, Walther K, Nikolaus M, Schrading S (2017) Impact of preoperative breast MR imaging and MR-guided surgery on diagnosis and surgical outcome of women with invasive breast cancer with and without DCIS component. Radiology 284(3):645–655

Lee SJ, Trikha S, Moy L, Baron P, diFlorio RM, Green ED, Heller SL, Holbrook AI, Lewin AA, Lourenco AP, Niell BL, Slanetz PJ, Stuckey AR, Vincoff NS, Weinstein SP, Yepes MM, Newell MS, Expert Panel on Breast Imaging (2017) ACR appropriateness criteria® evaluation of nipple discharge. J Am Coll Radiol 14(5S):S138–S153

Li GZ, Wong SM, Lester S, Nakhlis F (2018) Evaluating the risk of underlying malignancy in patients with pathologic nipple discharge. Breast J 24(4):624–627

Lippa N, Hurtevent-Labrot G, Ferron S, Boisserie-Lacroix M (2015) Nipple discharge: the role of imaging. Diagn Interv Imaging 96(10):1017–1032

Lourenco AP, Moy L, Baron P, Didwania AD, diFlorio RM, Heller SL, Holbrook AI, Lewin AA, Mehta TS, Niell BL, Slanetz PJ, Stuckey AR, Tuscano DS, Vincoff NS, Weinstein SP, Newell MS, Expert Panel on Breast Imaging (2018) ACR appropriateness criteria® breast implant evaluation. J Am Coll Radiol 15(5S):13–25

McGuire KP et al (2011) MRI staging after neoadjuvant chemotherapy for breast cancer: does tumor biology affect accuracy. Ann Surg Oncol 18:3149–3154

Mukhtar RA et al (2013) Clinically meaningful tumor reduction rates vary by prechemotherapy MRI phenotype and tumor subtype in the I-SPY 1 TRIAL (CALGB 150007/150012; ACRIN 6657). Ann Surg Oncol 20:3823–3830

National Comprehensive Cancer Network (2018) Breast cancer (Version 1.2018). http://www.nccn.org/professionals/physician_gls/pdf/breast.pdf. Accessed 16 May 2018

Nguyen C, Kettler MD, Swirsky ME, Miller VI, Scott C, Krause R, Hadro JA (2013) Male breast disease: pictorial review with radiologic-pathologic correlation. Radiographics 33:763–779

Niell BL, Lourenco AP, Moy L, Baron P, Didwania AD, diFlorio-Alexander RM, Heller SL, Holbrook AI, Le-Petross HT, Lewin AA, Mehta TS, Slanetz PJ, Stuckey AR, Tuscano DS, Ulaner GA, Vincoff NS, Weinstein SP, Newell MS (2018) ACR appropriateness criteria evaluation of the symptomatic male breast. J Am Coll Radiol 15:313–320

Panzironi G, Pediconi F, Sardanelli F (2019) Nipple discharge: the state of the art. BJR Open 1(1): 20180016

Patel BK, Ferraro C, Kosiorek HE, Loving VA, D'Orsi C, Newell M, Gray RJ (2018) Nipple discharge: imaging variability among U.S. radiologists. AJR Am J Roentgenol 211(4):920–925

Paula IB, Campos AM (2017) Breast imaging in patients with nipple discharge. Radiol Bras 50(6):383–388

Scaranelo AM, Marques AF, Smialowski EB, Lederman HM (2004) Evaluation of the rupture of silicone breast implants by mammography, ultrasonography and magnetic resonance imaging in asymptomatic patients: correlation with surgical findings. Sao Paulo Med J 122(2):41–47

Scheel JR et al (2018) MRI, clinical examination, and mammography for preoperative assessment of residual disease and pathologic complete response after neoadjuvant chemotherapy for breast cancer: ACRIN 6657 trial. AJR 210(6):1376–1385

Seiler SJ, Sharma PB, Hayes JC, Ganti R, Mootz AR, Eads ED, Teotia SS, Evans WP (2017) Multimodality imaging-based evaluation of single-lumen sili-cone breast implants for rupture. Radiographics 37(2):366–382

Shin K, Martaindale S, Whitman GJ (2018) Male breast magnetic resonance imaging: when is it helpful? Our experience over the last decade. Curr Probl Diagn Radiol (in press), accepted manuscript. Available online 10 Jan. pii: S0363-0188(17)30307-9

Thiruchelvam P, Walker JN, Rose K, Lewis J, Al-Mufti R (2016) Gynaecomastia. BMJ 354:i4833

Yang N, Muradali D (2011) The augmented breast: a pictorial review of the abnormal and unusual. Am J Roentgenol 196(4):451–460

Youn I et al (2015) Ultrasonography-guided surgical clip placement for tumor localization in patients undergoing neoadjuvant chemotherapy. J Breast Cancer 8(1):44–49

# Value-Based Radiology in Pediatric Imaging

Daniela Pinto and Sílvia Costa Dias

## Contents

D. Pinto (✉) · S. C. Dias
Department of Diagnostic and Interventional Radiology, University Hospital Centro Hospitalar São João, Porto, Portugal
e-mail: danielapintu@gmail.com

## Abstract

Based on five case scenarios encompassing common clinical questions in pediatric radiology the added value achieved through radiological expertise input will be highlighted. Clinic algorithms help in the imaging management of infants and children with urinary tract infection, like avoidance of urgent imaging in simple urinary tract infection. The scenarios address situations where the radiologist could help improve the outcomes, like the use of contrast-enhanced voiding urosonography as an alternative to voiding cystourethrogram, in detecting alterations in the urinary tract without the use of ionizing radiation. A case of pneumonia complicated with empyema highlights that ultrasound is the best method in the diagnosis and characterization of pleural effusions and can detect lung consolidation, necrotizing pneumonia and abscess (avoiding computed tomography in some cases). Pediatric cervical lymphadenopathies are common and radiologists can add value identifying the lymph nodes with suspicious US features that should prompt biopsy, helping in a faster diagnosis and reducing unnecessary follow-up US. A case of suspected appendicitis with a non-visualized appendix on US illustrates the added value of reporting the absence or presence of appendiceal secondary signs.

Med Radiol Diagn Imaging (2019)
https://doi.org/10.1007/174_2019_214, © Springer Nature Switzerland AG
Published Online: 02 July 2019

# 1 Introduction

"Children are not just small adults" is a well-worn phrase in the pediatric field. They have unique diseases and some diseases children might have in common with adults may have a different diagnostic approach. A great emphasis is given on ultrasound (US) in this chapter because we believe that its diagnostic capacity should be maximized in the pediatric population. Concern has increased about the risks of radiation exposure, specifically regarding a small but significant increase in the lifetime risk of fatal cancer in children who have undergone computed tomography (CT) exams. For other side, magnetic resonance imaging (MRI) is not widely available and, when available, its role is more relevant and relatively well established in brain, oncologic and musculoskeletal imaging. This chapter also focuses on updated guidelines and recommendations that help both radiologists and clinicians when facing similar scenarios to decide the best diagnostic approach with as little potential harm and cost as possible. Our five selected cases are resumed in Table 1.

# 2 Urinary Tract Infection

An 11-month-old female infant comes to the emergency department (ED) with unexplained fever of 38.5 °C. Urgent microscopic analysis of urine is positive for pyuria. A febrile UTI is correctly regarded as the most likely diagnosis and the antibiotic treatment is immediately started.

## 2.1 Role of Imaging: A Value-Based Approach

A common imaging request in this scenario is a renal and bladder US, either during the next days of inpatient stay for IV therapy or during the acute emergency episode of care. But, first of all we should divide UTIs in three different categories: typical, atypical, and recurrent as shown in Table 2.

Secondly, three different age groups should be kept in mind: 0–5, 6–35, and ≥36 months, as there are different recommendations also based on the age of the patient (Table 3).

**Table 1** Case scenarios to be displayed in this chapter

| Case | Issue | Key points |
|---|---|---|
| Case 1 | Urinary tract infection (UTI) | • Urgent ultrasound imaging is not indicated in typical or simple UTI |
| Case 2 | Postnatal imaging management of antenatally detected urinary tract dilation (UTD) | • Structured reports based on standard UTD classification system facilitates communication and helps in management<br>• Contrast-enhanced voiding urosonography (ceVUS) is an alternative to voiding cystourethrogram (VCUG) |
| Case 3 | Pneumonia complicated by empyema | • US as the preferred method to confirm and characterize parapneumonic effusions, providing additional valuable information regarding loculation with patient mobilization and parenchymal evaluation<br>• Clinical factors and imaging findings combined will define the best treatment, not just US findings such as septations<br>• CT should be reserved for complex cases and should not be performed routinely |
| Case 4 | Incidental cervical lymphadenopathy with suspicious features on US | • Cervical lymphadenopathy with suspicious features detected incidentally during US should always lead to a detailed thyroid examination, especially in an adolescent girl<br>• Increased risk of malignancy in pediatric thyroid nodules compared to adults |
| Case 5 | Non-visualized appendix on US in children with suspected appendicitis | • The absence of secondary signs when the appendix is not visualized on US has a high negative predictive value for appendicitis and should represent a negative study instead of "non-diagnostic" |

**Table 2** The three different categories of UTIs in pediatric age (based on British National Institute for Clinical Excellence (NICE) guideline 2018a)

| | Typical | Atypical | Recurrent |
|---|---|---|---|
| Features | – Absent atypical features<br>– Not recurrent | – Seriously ill (cf. National Institute for Clinical Excellence 2018b)<br>– Poor urine flow or raised creatinine<br>– Abdominal or bladder mass<br>– Antibiotic failure (within 48 h after starting)<br>– Infection with organisms other than *E. coli* | – ≥2 episodes of UTI with acute pyelonephritis/upper UTI, or<br>– 1 episode of UTI with acute pyelonephritis/upper UTI **plus** ≥1 episode of UTI with cystitis/lower UTI, or<br>– ≥3 episodes of UTI with cystitis/lower UTI |

**Table 3** Appropriate use criteria: ultrasound scan in UTI according to patient age (based on National Institute for Clinical Excellence 2018a)

| Test | Simple UTI/ responds well within 48 h | Atypical UTI | Recurrent UTI |
|---|---|---|---|
| *0–5 Months* | | | |
| US during acute infection | No | **Yes** | **Yes** |
| US within 6 weeks | **Yes** | No | No |
| *6–35 Months* | | | |
| US during acute infection | No | **Yes** | No |
| US within 6 weeks | No | No | **Yes** |
| *≥36 Months* | | | |
| US during acute infection | No | **Yes** | No |
| US within 6 weeks | No | No | **Yes** |

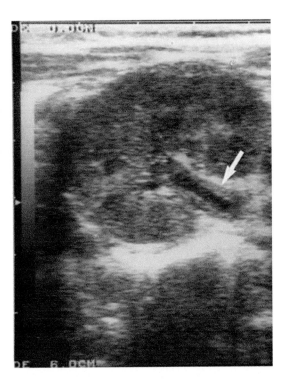

**Fig. 1** Thickening of the renal pelvis wall (arrow) and mild dilation in a companion case of pediatric acute pyelonephritis [Reprinted by permission from Springer Nature: Avni F.E., Hall M., Cassart M., Massez A. (2008) Urinary Tract Infection. In: Fotter R. (eds) Pediatric Uroradiology. Medical Radiology (Diagnostic Imaging). Springer, Berlin, Heidelberg]

## 2.2 Rationale

As we can see from the table above, only atypical UTI (any age) and recurrent UTI (in infants under 6 months) are indications for urgent US. This is in concordance with the American Academy of Pediatrics (AAP) position (American Academy of Pediatrics 2011) which states that only when the UTI is unusually clinically severe or substantial improvement is not occurring during the first 2 days of treatment then a renal and bladder US should be recommended. Performing a renal US in every single case of UTI could be misleading, because it can show a regular dilation produced by *E. coli* endotoxin that could be confused with a true structural hydronephrosis or obstruction (Fig. 1).

That is the reason why only if the infant is less than 6 months, should he or she have an US performed within 6 weeks after a simple UTI, to allow the possible infectious renal pelvic dilation to resolve and discard or confirm if true structural hydronephrosis (HDN) might have gone unnoticed in the prenatal obstetric imaging. So, the NICE guidelines tend to be more objective than those from AAP as they provide guidance on what signs and symptoms must be considered when a child is said to be "seriously ill" (National Institute for Clinical Excellence 2018b). NICE also provides guidance on when to request scintigraphy scan (DMSA) and VCUG. Briefly, the DMSA scan is indicated 4–6 months after the infection in case of an atypical UTI (until the age of 35 months) or recurrent UTI (any age). VCUG is indicated after the infection is treated only in case of an atypical or recurrent UTI until the age of 5 months (between the ages of 6 and 35 months it should be considered if some additional features are present) (National Institute for Clinical Excellence 2018a).

> **Key Points**
> - **Urgent ultrasound imaging**: is not indicated in typical or simple UTI.
> - **In typical or simple UTI**: consider ultrasound only in infants less than 6 months, and within the next 6 weeks after the UTI episode, to prevent misleading false positive cases of structural HDN.
> - **Benchmark/internal institutional audits**: should be performed to check normal or misleading US rates as some pediatricians resistant to change or not aware of guidelines might abuse on calling "atypical" or "seriously ill" in the request forms.

# 3    Postnatal Imaging Management of Antenatally Detected Urinary Tract Dilation

A term male newborn was noted to have unilateral left UTD on prenatal US with an anterior-posterior renal pelvic diameter (APRPD) of 10 mm. After birth, two US examinations were performed (one within the first 3 days of life and the other within 1 month of

age) that demonstrated an APRPD of 7 mm on the right kidney, and an APRPD of 11 mm on the left kidney with associated central calyceal dilatation. Additionally, mild bilateral dilatation was noted on both distal ureters. The bladder had normal wall thickness, absence of ureteroceles and emptied after voiding (Fig. 2). A VCUG was requested by the pediatric nephrologist to rule out vesicoureteral reflux (VUR) and posterior urethral valves (PUV). Nevertheless, the clinician decided to discuss this case in advance with the attending pediatric radiologist, who proposed to alternatively perform a ceVUS. The ceVUS showed bilateral grade II VUR (low grade), either with a fully distended bladder and during cyclic voiding. The urethra was also evaluated, during voiding, by a transperineal interscrotal approach that showed no valves, diverticula, and strictures (Fig. 3).

## 3.1    Role of Imaging: A Value-Based Approach

All newborns with a history of antenatal UTD should undergo a postnatal US evaluation. It is recommended to delay the first postnatal US at least 48 h after birth (because neonatal dehydration could underestimate the severity of hydronephrosis) except for cases of oligohydramnios, suspected urethral obstruction, and bilateral high-grade dilatation (Wiener and O'Hara 2002). The etiology of antenatal UTD includes transient dilation of the collecting system, upper/lower urinary tract obstructive uropathy, and nonobstructive processes such as vesicoureteral reflux. When UTD is observed on the postnatal US, approximately 49% of the children have VUR, compared with less than 5% when two postnatal US evaluations are normal (Ismaili et al. 2002). Currently, there is no clear evidence to support or to avoid postnatal imaging to diagnose VUR. The reason is because there is no compelling evidence that, in children with VUR, antibiotic prophylaxis would reduce the risk of recurrent UTI, and surgery does not provide neither a systematic

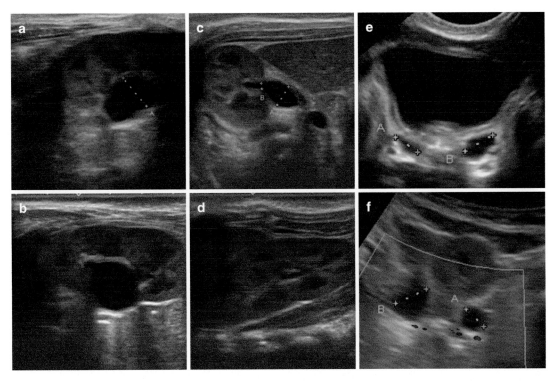

**Fig. 2** US performed 1 month after birth. (**a**) Axial image of the left kidney showing an APRPD of 11 mm. (**b**) Sagittal image of left kidney demonstrating central but not peripheral calyceal dilation. The renal parenchyma is normal. (**c**) Axial image of the right kidney showing an APRPD of 3 mm on the hilum and 7 mm in the extrarenal pelvis. (**d**) Sagittal image of right kidney demonstrating neither central nor peripheral calyceal dilation. The renal parenchyma is normal. (**e**) Axial image of the bladder with normal parietal thickness and mildly dilated distal ureters. (**f**) Axial image showing again dilated distal ureters, and the bladder after voiding

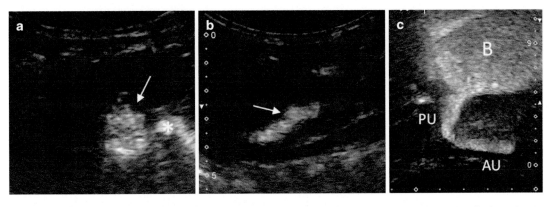

**Fig. 3** ceVUS images during voiding at 2 months of age. (**a**) Sagittal image showing contrast in the left renal pelvis (arrow) and proximal ureter (asterisk) corresponding to grade II VUR. (**b**) Sagittal image showing contrast in the central calyceal system on the right kidney (arrow) also corresponding to grade II VUR. (**c**) Sagittal image (anatomic orientation) with a transperineal interscrotal approach nicely depicting a normal urethra (*PU* posterior urethra, *AU* anterior urethra, *B* bladder)

reduction in UTI nor a reduction in the development of renal damage (Nagler et al. 2011). The latest multidisciplinary consensus on the classification of prenatal and postnatal urinary tract dilation (UTD Classification System), created by representatives from eight societies, proposed a risk-based postnatal management of UTD (Nguyen et al. 2014). In Table 4, the postnatal risk stratification groups based on six US findings are presented, and in Table 5 the proposed imaging studies and therapeutic management for each group is presented.

According to this new classification, VCUG is just truly recommended on UTD P3 (high risk). Our patient had an UTD P2 (intermediate risk) in the left kidney—an ARPD of 11 mm, but with abnormal ureters (the panel recommends that stratification of risk should be based on the grading of UT dilation in the most severely affected side). The clinical hypothesis of PUV raised by the pediatric nephrologist is very unlikely because there is no peripheral calyceal dilatation on either side and the kidneys and bladder are otherwise normal. In this context, a further investigation for VUR is not mandatory, though it is still reasonable or good practice to just perform the recommended US follow-up. For low risk and intermediate risk cases, recommendations for evaluation with VCUG are left to the discretion of the clinician. Nevertheless, we should keep in mind that children are particularly at risk for the adverse effects of ionizing radiation. When available, ceVUS should be considered as an alternative option to the current gold standard, VCUG. Although both diagnostic procedures require catheterization, ceVUS provides high quality diagnostic images that allow the urinary tract to be evaluated without the use of ionizing radiation. In a recent literature review (Chua et al. 2019), it was verified that the diagnostic accuracy of ceVUS in diagnosing VUR among children is comparable to VCUG, specifically for high-grade VUR and in younger children. Additionally, ceVUS is able to evaluate the urethra and to exclude underlying pathology that includes posterior or anterior valves, diverticula, and strictures (Duran et al. 2017).

**Table 4** UTD Risk Stratification—Postnatal Presentation for UTD P1 (low risk), UTD P2 (intermediate risk), and UTD P3 (high risk)

|  | Normal | UTD P1 | UTD P2 | UTD P3 |
|---|---|---|---|---|
| APRPD | <10 mm | ≥10–14 mm | ≥15 mm | ≥15 mm |
| Calyceal dilatation | None/central | Central | Peripheral | Peripheral |
| Parenchymal thickness | Normal | Normal | Normal | Abnormal |
| Parenchymal appearance | Normal | Normal | Normal | Abnormal |
| Ureters | Normal | Normal | Abnormal | Abnormal |
| Bladder | Normal | Normal | Normal | Abnormal |

Please note that stratification is based on the most concerning ultrasound finding. For example, if the APRPD is in the UTD P1 range, but there is peripheral calyceal dilation, the classification is UTD P2. If there is a ureteral dilation with an APRPD of 11 mm (as in our case scenario) the classification is UTD P2. The presence of parenchymal abnormalities denotes UTD P3 classification as long as there is any urinary tract dilation (Adapted from Nguyen et al. 2014)

**Table 5** Management schema based on UTD classification system risk stratification of UTD P1, UTD P2, and UTD P3 (Adapted from Nguyen et al. 2014)

|  | UTD P1 | UTD P2 | UTD P3 |
|---|---|---|---|
| Follow-up US | 1–6 months | 1–3 months | 1 month |
| VCUG | Physician's Discretion | Physician's Discretion | Recommended |
| Antibiotics | Physician's Discretion | Physician's Discretion | Recommended |
| Functional scan | Not recommended | Physician's Discretion | Physician's Discretion |

**Key Points**
- **Added value of UTD classification system**: It allows for the elaboration of a structured ultrasound report with standardized terminology that facilitates communication among providers and helps to decide the best management for all children (including avoiding unnecessary radiologic exams).
- **ceVUS as an alternative to VCUG**: If further evaluation of VUR is necessary we should keep in mind that ceVUS has a similar diagnostic accuracy when compared to VCUG but without ionizing radiation.

## 4 Pneumonia Complicated by Empyema

A 5-year-old female was first observed in the ED of an outside institution with a history of fever and vomits. The diagnosis of appendicitis was excluded and chest radiograph showed no consolidation. The child was discharged from the ED with reassurance and instructions to return. As the fever persisted, the child returned 3 days later, and this time she was admitted with the diagnosis of right-sided lobar pneumonia (Fig. 4a). On the third day of inpatient stay there was clinical deterioration besides empiric antibiotic therapy, with lab tests showing prominent leukocytosis $35 \times 10^9$/L (72% neutrophils) and a C-reactive protein of 300 mg/L. The child developed respiratory distress, with an oxygen supply need of 15 L/min. The chest radiograph showed a right white lung, suggesting a rapidly enlarging coexistent pleural effusion (Fig. 4b). The child was then transferred to our tertiary academic center. An US was requested to characterize the pleural effusion, revealing a large volume heterogeneous effusion with septations. Coexistent lung consolidation with air bronchogram was also depicted. The surgical team decided for a video-assisted thoracoscopic surgery (VATS), where lysis of adhesions, pleural decortication, and pus aspiration (positive for *S. pneumonia*) were performed. A first follow-up US showed some complex effusion and lung consolation with foci of necrotizing parenchyma

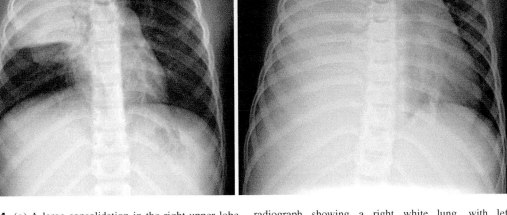

**Fig. 4** (**a**) A large consolidation in the right upper lobe and small one in the middle lobe were shown in the chest radiograph done at admission. (**b**) Bedside chest radiograph showing a right white lung, with left mediastinal shift suggesting a coexistent large right-sided pleural effusion

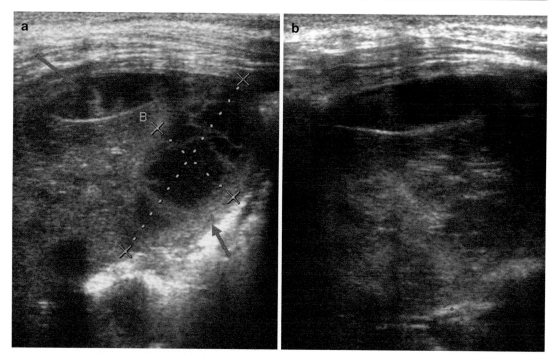

**Fig. 5** (**a, b**) Complex effusion (solid arrows) and necrotizing parenchymal foci (dotted arrows)

(Fig. 5). The child had good clinical response with improvement of the findings and no further effusion drainage was needed.

## 4.1 Role of Imaging: The Importance of Ultrasound

Current guidelines advocate that chest radiograph is not recommended routinely in children with uncomplicated community-acquired pneumonia, who are not hospital admitted for treatment (Harris et al. 2011; Andronikou et al. 2017a). The radiographic findings cannot accurately differentiate viral from bacterial infection. In our case scenario, an initial radiograph (at the ED) was performed and the child was not hospitalized thereafter, reflecting still a common clinical practice. In the Infectious Diseases Society of America (IDSA) guidelines (Bradley et al. 2011), chest radiographs with an additional lateral view should be obtained in all patient admitted for management of community-acquired pneumonia. An additional view is not, however, routinely recommended in the British Thoracic Society (BTS) guidelines (Harris et al. 2011). Follow-up chest radiograph is not required for a previously healthy child with a good clinical response. If a child remains feverish or unwell after 48 h of hospital admission, the suspicious of complication, such as a developing empyema, should be raised and reevaluation is necessary (Harris et al. 2011).

Ultrasound is the preferred method for identifying and characterizing parapneumonic effusions (Balfour-Lynn et al. 2005; Mong et al. 2012; Westra and Choy 2009). Ultrasound can estimate the volume of pleural effusion, being able to detect smaller volumes and distinguish between pleural fluid and underlying lung consolidation, which is particularly helpful in the white hemithorax (Calder and Owens 2009). Ultrasound has the ability to characterize pleural effusion as anechoic, with septations and echogenic component. Ultrasound shows superiority in the detection of fibrin strands versus CT (Kurian et al. 2009), resulting in a more accurate technique to differentiate complicated effusions

(Westra and Choy 2009), lacking ionizing radiation. However, caution has to be taken when distinguishing between exudates and transudates. Internally echogenic or septated effusions are almost always exudates, and transudates are usually anechoic. However, approximately one-third of exudates can also be anechoic (Calder and Owens 2009; Tomà and Owens 2013; Yang et al. 1992).

Ultrasound is also very valuable as a dynamic examination, being able to classify an effusion as free fluid or loculated, the latter meaning that the collection is unchanged with positional maneuvers (Calder and Owens 2009). Ultrasound is also useful in guiding thoracentesis or drain placement. In our case scenario we might query if an earlier sonographic evaluation could have been helpful, as detection of complex effusions might influence triage for treatment groups (Westra and Choy 2009). Nevertheless, radiologists should be aware that the treatment decision of drainage is not to be defined by imaging alone, it is a combined approach—effusions that are enlarging and/or compromising respiratory function should not be managed with antibiotic therapy only (Balfour-Lynn et al. 2005). In IDSA guidelines, the volume of the effusion is an important factor, with large effusions influencing management for drainage. An effusion in a persistently feverish child is also an indication for drainage (Harris et al. 2011).

Regarding the management approach for pleural effusion drainage, there are different possibilities like simple tube drainage, tube drainage with fibrinolytics or VATS. It is advised that children who require chest tube drainage should be transferred to a tertiary care center.

## 4.2 Role of Imaging: Is CT Really Needed?

This is a very important question. At some point it may be arguable, but the medical team should discuss this issue, oriented to each specific case. Pleural and lung ultrasound (Cox et al. 2017), and specifically lung ultrasound for the diagnosis of pneumonia (Stadler et al. 2017), are current hot topics in radiology. In our case scenario, lung parenchymal complications, such as necrotizing pneumonia (NP), could occur, but weren't detected in the first ultrasound. So radiologists should be aware that ultrasound may detect parenchymal abnormalities and examine the parenchymal consolidation (also with Doppler evaluation), although it could be more time consuming. Valuable information can be added to the radiograph investigation, when looking for necrotizing foci or, more rarely, an abscess. NP incidence is increasing (Spencer and Thomas 2014), with *Streptococcus pneumonia* as the predominant agent. Children with NP have an increased risk for developing a bronchopleural fistula (Sawicki et al. 2008).

The detection of suppurative pleural and parenchymal complications is important for the length of antibiotic therapy and may also interfere with other treatment choices (Andronikou et al. 2017b).

Kurian et al. (Kurian et al. 2009) in their series found that chest ultrasound provided similar data to CT in the assessment of lung consolidation, lung necrosis, and abscess. Contrast-enhanced CT is preferred over non-contrast CT to show parenchymal complications, being a very sensitive and accurate method. Nevertheless, CT is, in most cases, unnecessary for the management of empyema and should not be performed routinely (Balfour-Lynn et al. 2005). CT has a role in complex cases, being useful for evaluating advanced parenchymal disease, chest drain position, drainage or medical treatment failure and, with a particularly relevance, in immunocompromised children. When surgery is the selected treatment, some surgeons request a preoperative CT scan (Calder and Owens 2009). Suspect of abscess or NP is often raised on chest radiographs, and contrast-enhanced CT can confirm these findings (Harris et al. 2011); however it does not justify its routine use in pleuropulmonary infections in general (Tomà and Owens 2013). CT may also be valuable when other modalities are inconclusive, and in complex cases as a "road-map"

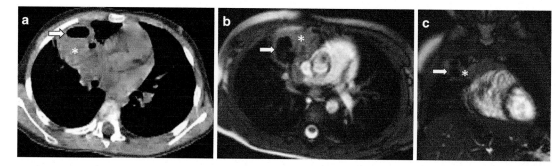

**Fig. 6** (**a**, **b**) Images from a companion case of a 5-year-old girl with cavitary pneumonia. (**a**) CT image shows right upper lobe consolidation (asterisk) surrounding a cavity containing an air-fluid level (arrow). (**b**) Axial non-enhanced T2-weighted balanced fast field echo MR image (TR: 3 ms, TE: 2 ms, flip angle: 60°) shows right upper lobe consolidation (asterisk) surrounding an air-filled cavity (arrow). (**c**) Coronal non-enhanced T2-weighted balanced fast field echo MR image (TR: 4 ms, TE: 2 ms, flip angle: 60°) shows right upper lobe consolidation (asterisk) surrounding an air-filled cavity (arrow) [Reprinted by permission from Springer Nature: Liszewski, M.C., Görkem, S., Sodhi, K.S. et al. Pediatr Radiol (2017) 47: 1420. https://doi.org/10.1007/s00247-017-3865-2]

examination (Calder and Owens 2009; Tomà and Owens 2013). This was not critical in our case for the surgical approach, as the patient was submitted directly to VATS. The postoperative complex effusion detected by ultrasound did not require additional drainage.

As imaging technology is advancing in a fast pace, MRI has already proved to be another accurate alternative for the evaluation of complicated pneumonia. Alterations such as consolidation, ground glass opacities, parenchyma necrosis, abscess, pleural effusion, and empyema can be nicely depicted on MRI (Attenberger et al. 2014; Peprah et al. 2012; Peltola et al. 2008; Gorkem et al. 2013). Necrosis can be evidenced by foci of hypointense signal typically within an area of pulmonary consolidation that shows hyperintensity on T2-weighted MRI. Locules of air can also be shown on pulmonary necrosis. Rounded non-enhancing foci of signal abnormality surrounded by a rim of hyperenhancing pulmonary consolidation, showing inner hyperintensity on T2-weighted images, and restricted diffusion on diffusion-weighted images put into evidence the presence of pulmonary abscess (Liszewski et al. 2017). Pulmonary abscess may also contain an air-fluid level or be completely air-filled. The air-containing regions (either in necrosis or in abscess) lack signal on all MRI sequences (Fig. 6).

**Key Points**

- **Ultrasound**: is the preferred method to confirm and characterize parapneumonic effusions. Loculation detection with patient mobilization and parenchymal evaluation using this technique may provide valuable information.
- **CT should not be routinely performed**: this technique should be reserved for more complex cases.

## 5 Incidental Cervical Lymphadenopathy with Suspicious Features on US

A 14-year-old female, with a history of previous excised schwannoma of the mentum was appointed for a follow-up cervical ultrasound in our department. The adolescent had no other relevant clinical history and was asymptomatic. A suspicious cervical lymph node was detected on the right middle internal jugular chain (level III), with loss of normal architecture, absent fatty hilum, a cystic component and some small punctate echogenic foci, suggesting microcalcifications (Fig. 7).

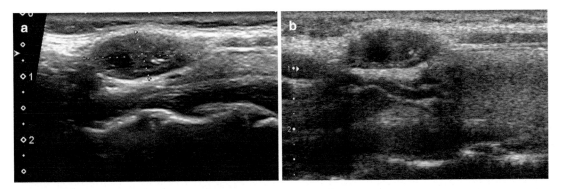

**Fig. 7** (**a, b**) Lymphadenopathy with 17 × 8 mm with cystic component (solid arrow) and some microcalcifications (dotted arrow)

Due to suspicious findings and also to the location of the lymph node, the thyroid gland was carefully examined (the cervical examination was repeated, being performed by three different persons, including one radiology resident and two consultant radiologists) and neither thyroid abnormalities were detected on physical examination nor thyroid nodules were identified at US. No other lymphadenopathies or cervical abnormalities were depicted. A fine needle aspiration (FNA) biopsy of the lymph node was recommended and performed, revealing a papillary carcinoma lymph node metastasis. Total thyroidectomy was later performed, with right modified radical neck dissection, revealing a right lower pole papillary carcinoma with 1 × 2 × 2 mm maximal diameters and ill-defined margins. No other thyroid lesions were present. From the 26 lymph nodes excised 4 were metastatic. The final pathology report revealed a papillary carcinoma, follicular variant, pT1a N1b.

## 5.1 Rationale

Pediatric cervical lymphadenopathy is a very common finding in clinical practice, being responsible for a significant volume of ultrasound examinations. The majority of the clinically detected cervical lymphadenopathies are related to benign and self-limited inflammatory processes.

The clinical history, the physical examination, the reevaluation after treatment, and lab tests will determine if imaging is necessary. The adult size criteria for cervical lymphadenopathy are also applied for children (Nolder 2013).

Hard, nonmobile, and painless lymph nodes are suspicious clinical findings, as well as progressive nodal enlargement and no response to treatment, or the presence of systemic symptoms (Ludwig et al. 2012). Other findings suspicious for malignancy are large lymph node size (>2 cm), multiple sites of lymphadenopathy (>2), and supraclavicular location (Nolder 2013). If there are clinical concerns for cervical lymph nodes, ultrasound will be the first line examination. Cervical involvement is more usual in Hodgkin's lymphoma than in non-Hodgkin lymphoma, with more common involvement of the internal jugular and spinal accessory nodes. Ultrasound findings may reveal enlarged lymph nodes or may form a conglomerate, being usually homogenous and hypoechoic (Siegel 2019). Bilateral involvement is common and calcifications are mainly a posttreatment feature. Metastatic lymphadenopathy in children is usually from head and neck rhabdomyosarcoma and less commonly thyroid carcinoma and neuroblastoma. Ultrasound features of malignant lymphadenopathy are round (loss of the normal ovoid shape), hypoechoic, absent hilum and irregular margins (Siegel 2019). Kumbhar et al. (2016), in the context of differentiated thyroid cancer, describe as suspicious findings for metastatic lymph nodes the presence of microcalcifications, cystic degeneration, increased peripheral vascularity, echogenicity greater than adjacent muscle, rounded morphology, and loss of the fatty hilum. Microcalcifications and cystic degeneration have the highest specificity of all ultrasound features predictive of malignant involvement (Kumbhar et al. 2016; Haugen et al. 2016).

There are specific guidelines for children with thyroid nodules and differentiated thyroid cancer (Francis et al. 2015), resulting from clinical, histological, and genetic differences. Thyroid nodules are uncommon in children comparing to adults. However, they have a much higher incidence of malignancy—one in four nodules will be malignant in children (Essenmacher et al. 2017). Adolescent girls have a tenfold higher risk compared to younger children, with a female:male distribution of 5:1 in adolescence (Francis et al. 2015). In pediatric thyroid cancer there is a higher risk of lymph node metastasis, extra-thyroid extension and pulmonary metastasis at the time of diagnosis. Although the disease commonly manifests in a more advanced stage in children, the prognosis is comparatively favorable (Essenmacher et al. 2017). The threshold for FNA biopsy in thyroid nodules children is lower, regarding the clinical context and in the presence of ultrasound suspicious findings, with less emphasis on size criterion. Another significant difference is that 30% of hyperfunctioning nodules in nuclear scintigraphy will be malignant, so surgery is recommended without biopsy. There is also another unique difference in children: the papillary thyroid cancer may present as diffuse infiltrating disease, with diffuse enlargement of one lobe or the whole gland (Francis et al. 2015), which may justify FNA biopsy if the appearance is suspicious. If a fine needle aspiration biopsy is indeterminate, surgery is recommended.

In our case, it was the ultrasound findings of the lymph node that claimed our attention. Even without any thyroid nodule detected or other cervical findings, we were concerned and recommended directly the FNA biopsy, resulting in a prompt diagnosis.

**Key Points**
- **Incidental suspicious cervical lymphadenopathy**: when detected during ultrasound, always perform a detailed thyroid examination, especially in an adolescent girl.
- **Higher risk of malignancy in pediatric thyroid nodules**: there is an increased risk of malignancy in the pediatric population compared to adults, with several other specificities. The radiologist should be aware of the pediatric guidelines to approach this issue.

## 6 Case 5: Non-visualized Appendix on US in Children with Suspected Appendicitis

A 9-year-old boy presented to the ED with one episode of vomit and acute abdominal pain. He had no diarrhea or fever. Clinical examination revealed a soft abdomen with tenderness and guarding in the right lower quadrant. An US was requested to rule out appendicitis but the appendix was not identified. In the US report the radiologist declared no free fluid, no fluid collections, no hyperechoic mesenteric fat, and no dilated small bowel loops. The final impression on the report was "no US features of appendicitis". Blood tests were unremarkable. The patient stayed in the ED for observation and he was discharged with complete resolution of symptoms six hours later. Seven months later he visited again the ED with acute abdominal pain. At this time, the US depicted a normal appendix, with no positive findings elsewhere in the pelvis or abdomen.

### 6.1 Role of Imaging: A Value-Based Approach

The clinical suspicion of appendicitis is the main cause for a child to undergo an abdominal ultrasound in the ED. Ultrasound is the preferred initial imaging study in this context for obvious reasons (absence of radiation, no need for sedation and low cost). In a meta-analysis (Doria et al. 2006), its sensitivity and specificity to diagnose appendicitis in the pediatric population have been reported to be approximately 90%. A large prospective study showed that, at US, a thick noncompressible appendix with maximum outer wall diameter (MOD) greater than 6 mm has 98% sensitivity and specificity of being positive for acute appendicitis (Kaiser et al. 2002). Additionally, the most accurate periappendiceal finding for appendicitis is the presence of inflammatory fat changes, with a negative predictive value of 91% and a positive predictive value of 76% (Kaiser et al. 2002). Other studies, only focusing on the pediatric population, advocate that a 7.5 mm MOD threshold may be more optimal for diagnosing appendicitis when secondary signs are absent or in equivocal studies (Fallon et al. 2015; Goldin et al. 2011).

The proportion of a non-visualized appendix (NVA) on ultrasound can be as high as 76% when the study is performed outside of tertiary care centers (Held et al. 2018). Historically, when the appendix was not seen, US was considered "non-diagnostic" for acute appendicitis. Nevertheless, there are several studies in the pediatric population demonstrating that a NVA on US has a high negative predictive value (NPV) for appendicitis (92–100%) in the absence of secondary signs (Held et al. 2018; Binkovitz et al. 2015; Cohen et al. 2015; Nah et al. 2017; Larson et al. 2015; Wiersma et al. 2009). The secondary signs considered vary among studies but they all include thickened echogenic mesenteric fat in the right lower quadrant and extraluminal fluid collection. Other signs included are free fluid/pericecal fluid and local dilated small bowel loop. The presence of a small amount of free fluid in the pelvis in postpubertal girls should not be considered a secondary sign. A large study by Cohen et al. (2015) also analyzed other predictors for acute appendicitis such as the white blood cell count (WBC) count. They demonstrated that in patients with WBC $<7.5 \times 10^9/L$, a non-visualized appendix has a NPV of 98.86%.

There is discrepancy in the literature if obesity reduces the accuracy of US in the pediatric population when appendicitis is suspected—or not. Sometimes the visualization of the right lower quadrant in obese children is suboptimal but the radiologist should mention it on the exam report whenever he or she does not feel comfortable to exclude imaging features of appendicitis.

Our case scenario is one of the many cases that a non-visualized appendix without secondary signs of appendicitis on US is a true negative finding. A structured US report (Fig. 8) describing not only the appendix but also the secondary signs reduces the number of equivocal or "non-diagnostic" studies and helps to avoid further diagnostic imaging (Fallon et al. 2015; Binkovitz et al. 2015).

---

**Key Points**

- **Reduce equivocal reports**: The presence or absence of secondary findings of appendicitis should always be mentioned on the US report.
- **Increase value, reduce costs**: The absence of secondary signs when the appendix is not visualized has a high negative predictive value for appendicitis and should represent a negative study instead of "non-diagnostic."

---

## 7 Summary

We hope the reader had a good in-depth understanding from the presented case scenarios, so one can translate the gained input to everyday life, with the ultimate goal of providing the best and most valuable care not only to the children but also to the family or related caregivers.

As the expertise input from the pediatric radiologist is pivotal for the selection of the best imaging exam to be done, the radiologist's perspective should be taken into account in the multidisciplinary discussions or when on call in the emergency shift. Pediatric patients should be imaged wisely and gently. Radiation matters.

**a**

EXAM: Limited abdominal ultrasound

CLINICAL HISTORY: [Abdominal pain – concern for appendicitis]

PRIOR STUDIES: [None]

FINDINGS:

Appendix:
-Visualized: [Completely]
-Fluid-filled: [Yes]
-Compressible: [No]
-Maximum diameter with compression (outer wall to outer wall): [11 mm]
-Appendicolith: [No]
-Wall
  --Hyperemia: [No]
  --Thickening (>2 mm): [Yes]
  --Loss of mural stratification: [Yes]

Free fluid: [No]

Increased echogenicity of periappendiceal fat: [Yes]

Abscess: [No]

Additional findings: [None]

IMPRESSION:

Appendicitis score: 5a

Alternative/additional diagnosis: [None]

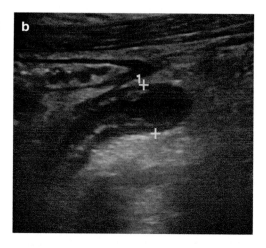

**Fig. 8** (**a**) An example of structured reporting template. Values for the fields in red can be changed at the discretion of the interpreting radiologist. (**b**) Gray-scale US image of surgically proven non-perforated acute appendicitis, in a companion case, with a diameter of 1.1 cm, wall thickening, loss of mural stratification, and increased echogenicity of periappendiceal fat [Reprinted by permission from Springer Nature: Fallon, S.C., Orth, R.C., Guillerman, R.P. et al. Pediatr Radiol (2015) 45: 1945. https://doi.org/10.1007/s00247-015-3443-4]

# References

American Academy of Pediatrics (2011) Steering committee on quality improvement, subcommittee on urinary tract infection: urinary tract infection: clinical practice guideline for the diagnosis and management of the initial UTI in febrile infants and children 2 to 24 months. Pediatrics 128:595–610

Andronikou S, Lambert E, Halton J et al (2017a) Guidelines for the use of chest radiographs in community-acquired pneumonia in children and adolescents. Pediatr Radiol 47:1405–1411

Andronikou S, Goussard P, Sorantin E (2017b) Computed tomography in children with community-acquired pneumonia. Pediatr Radiol 47:1431–1440

Attenberger UI, Morelli JN, Henzler T et al (2014) 3 Tesla proton MRI for the diagnosis of pneumonia/lung infiltrates in neutropenic patients with acute myeloid leukemia: initial results in comparison to HRCT. Eur J Radiol 83:e61–e66

Balfour-Lynn IM, Abrahamson E, Cohen G et al (2005) BTS guidelines for the management of pleural infection in children. Thorax 60(Suppl I):i1–i21

Binkovitz LA, Unsdorfer KML, Thapa P et al (2015) Pediatric appendiceal ultrasound: accuracy, determinacy and clinical outcomes. Pediatr Radiol 45:1934

Bradley JS, Byington CL, Shah SS et al (2011) The management of community-acquired pneumonia infants and children older than 3 months of age: clinical practice guidelines by the Pediatric Infectious Diseases Society and the Infectious Diseases Society of America. Clin Infect Dis 53(7):e25–e76

Calder A, Owens CM (2009) Imaging of parapneumonic pleural effusions and empyema in children. Pediatr Radiol 39:527–537

Chua ME, Kim JK, Mendoza JS, Fernandez N, Ming JM, Marson A, Lorenzo AJ, Lopes RI, Takahashi MS (2019) The evaluation of vesicoureteral reflux among children using contrast enhanced ultrasound: a literature review. J Pediatr Urol 15:12–17. https://doi.org/10.1016/j.jpurol.2018.11.006

Cohen B, Bowling J, Midulla P et al (2015) The non-diagnostic ultrasound in appendicitis: is a non-visualized appendix the same as a negative study? J Pediatr Surg 50(6):923–927

Cox M, Soudack M, Podberesky DJ et al (2017) Pediatric chest ultrasound: a practical approach. Pediatr Radiol 47:1058–1068

Doria AS, Moineddin R, Kellenberger CJ et al (2006) US or CT for diagnosis of appendicitis in children and adults? A meta-analysis. Radiology 241:83–94

Duran C, Beltrán VP, González A, Gómez C, Riego JD (2017) Contrast-enhanced voiding urosonography for vesicoureteral reflux diagnosis in children. Radiographics 37(6):1854–1869. https://doi.org/10.1148/rg.2017170024

Essenmacher AC, Joyce PH Jr, Kao SC et al (2017) Sonographic evaluation of pediatric thyroid nodules. Radiographics 37:1731–1752

Fallon SC, Orth RC, Guillerman RP et al (2015) Development and validation of an ultrasound scoring system for children with suspected acute appendicitis. Pediatr Radiol 45:1945

Francis GL, Waguespack SG, Bauer AJ et al (2015) Management guidelines for children with thyroid nodules and differentiated thyroid cancer. Thyroid 25(7):716–759

Goldin AB, Khanna P, Thapa M et al (2011) Revised ultrasound criteria for appendicitis in children improve diagnostic accuracy. Pediatr Radiol 41:993

Gorkem SB, Coskun A, Yikilmaz A et al (2013) Evaluation of pediatric thoracic disorders: comparison of unenhanced fastimaging-sequence 1.5-T MRI and contrast-enhanced MDCT. AJR Am J Roentgenol 200:1352–1357

Harris M, Clark J, Coote N et al (2011) British Thoracic Society guidelines for the management of community acquired pneumonia in children: update 2011. Thorax 66:ii1–ii23

Haugen BR, Alexander EK, Bible KC et al (2016) 2015 American Thyroid Association Management Guidelines for adult patients with thyroid nodules and differentiated thyroid cancer. The American Thyroid Association Guidelines Task Force on thyroid nodules and differentiated thyroid cancer. Thyroid 26(1):1–133

Held JM, McEvoy CS, Auten JD et al (2018) The nonvisualized appendix and secondary signs on ultrasound for pediatric appendicitis in the community hospital setting. Pediatr Surg Int 34:1287

Ismaili K, Avni FE, Hall M, Brussels Free University Perinatal Nephrology Study Group (2002) Results of systematic voiding cystourethrography in infants with antenatally diagnosed renal pelvis dilation. J Pediatr 141:21–24

Kaiser S, Frenckner B, Jorulf HK (2002) Suspected appendicitis in children: US and CT. A prospective randomized study. Radiology 223:633–638

Kumbhar SS, O'Malley RB, Robinson TJ et al (2016) Why thyroid surgeons are frustrated with radiologists: lessons learned pre- and postoperative US. Radiographics 36:2141–2153

Kurian J, Levin TL, Han BK (2009) Comparison of ultrasound and CT in the evaluation of pneumonia complicated by parapneumonic effusion in children. AJR 193:1648–1654

Larson DB, Trout AT, Fierke SF et al (2015) Improvement in diagnostic accuracy of ultrasound of the pediatric appendix through the use of equivocal interpretive categories. Am J Roentgenol 204:849–856

Liszewski MC, Görkem S, Sodhi KS et al (2017) Lung magnetic resonance imaging for pneumonia in children. Pediatr Radiol 47:1420. https://doi.org/10.1007/s00247-017-3865-2

Ludwig BJ, Wang J, Nadgir RN et al (2012) Imaging cervical lymphadenopathy in children and young adults. AJR 199:1105–1113

Mong A, Epelma M, Darge K (2012) Ultrasound of the pediatric chest. Pediatr Radiol 42:1287–1297

Nagler EV, Williams G, Hodson EM, Craig JC (2011) Interventions for primary vesicoureteric reflux. Cochrane Database Syst Rev (6):CD001532

Nah SA, Ong SS, Lim WX et al (2017) Clinical relevance of the nonvisualized appendix on ultrasonography of the abdomen in children. J Pediatr 182:164–169

National Institute for Clinical Excellence (2018a) Urinary tract infection in under 16s: diagnosis and management. Clinical guideline. nice.org.uk/guidance/cg54. Accessed 1 Jul 2018

National Institute for Clinical Excellence (2018b) Fever in under 5s: assessment and initial management. Clinical guideline. nice.org.uk/guidance/cg160. Accessed 1 Jul 2018

Nguyen HT, Benson CB, Bromley B et al (2014) Multidisciplinary consensus on the classification of prenatal and postnatal urinary tract dilation (UTD classification system). J Pediatr Urol 10:982–998

Nolder AR (2013) Paediatric cervical lymphadenopathy: when to biopsy? Curr Opin Otolaryngol Head Neck Surg 21:567–570

Peltola V, Ruuskanen O, Svedstrom E (2008) Magnetic resonance imaging of lung infections in children. Pediatr Radiol 38:1225–1231

Peprah KO, Andronikou S, Goussard P (2012) Characteristic magnetic resonance imaging low T2 signal intensity of necrotic lung parenchyma in children with pulmonary tuberculosis. J Thorac Imaging 27:171–174 33

Sawicki GS, Lu FL, Valim C et al (2008) Necrotizing pneumonia is an increasingly detected complication of pneumonia in children. Eur Respir J 31:1285–1291

Siegel MJ (2019) Pediatric sonography, 5th edn. Lippincott Williams & Wilkins (LWW), Philadelphia, PA, pp 132–133

Spencer DA, Thomas MF (2014) Necrotising pneumonia in children. Paediatr Respir Rev 15(3):240–2455

Stadler JA, Andronikou S, Zar H (2017) Lung ultrasound for the diagnosis of community-acquired pneumonia in children. Pediatr Radiol 47:1412–1419

Tomà P, Owens CM (2013) Chest ultrasound in children: critical appraisal. Pediatr Radiol 43:1427–1434

Westra SJ, Choy G (2009) What imaging should be performed for the diagnosis and management of pulmonar infections? Pediatr Radiol 39(Suppl 2):S178–S183

Wiener JS, O'Hara SM (2002) Optimal timing of initial postnatal ultrasonography in newborns with prenatal hydronephrosis. J Urol 168(4 Pt 2):1826–1829

Wiersma F, Toorenvliet B, Bloem J et al (2009) US examination of the appendix in children with suspected appendicitis: the additional value of secondary signs. Eur Radiol 19:455–461

Yang PC, Luh KT, Chang DB et al (1992) Value of sonography in determining the nature of pleural effusion: analysis of 320 cases. AJR 159:29–33

# Value-Based Radiology in Cardiovascular Imaging

Carlos Francisco Silva

## Contents

### Abstract

In this chapter six case scenarios are presented encompassing many common questions and issues that we may frequently face in the field of cardiovascular imaging and where the radiologists will bring added value through their expertise input. Scenarios like those where one can clearly improve patient outcomes are detailed, like the management of inferior vena cava (IVC) filter through a software that helps to track patients or through the implementation of specific macros for CT reading highlighting key points in IVC filter description. The added value for patient outcomes regarding coronary CTA is also highlighted, namely the help in early discharge from emergency department (ED) in the setting of chest pain of doubtful coronary origin. Also, scenarios where the radiologist can also add value, but mainly through helping to reduce redundancy or unnecessary imaging, that is in the end reducing the final healthcare costs are detailed, like the case for stress imaging in preoperative setting or venous thromboembolism, namely in the optimization of the diagnostic workup involving imaging tests.

C. F. Silva (✉)
Department of Diagnostic and Interventional
Radiology, University Hospital Heidelberg,
Heidelberg, Germany
e-mail: Carlos.dasilva@med.uni-heidelberg.de

Med Radiol Diagn Imaging (2019)
https://doi.org/10.1007/174_2018_205, © Springer Nature Switzerland AG
Published Online: 19 February 2019

# 1 Introduction

The field of cardiovascular imaging is ever evolving with continuous update of key information that should translate to practice if one wants to achieve the best value in the episode of care, either through increase in outcomes (the equation numerator) or through cost reduction (the equation denominator). Six cases, resumed in Table 1, are displayed with the purpose to give the reader a feeling of *déjá vu*, that is, real-world, common cases that we frequently came across in our work as radiologists or healthcare professionals, cases that have led us to question if that was really the best option, the best or the most appropriate imaging test. Answers and guidance with up-to-date best knowledge are provided.

# 2 Case 1: Deep Venous Thrombosis

A 23-year-old female presented with acute unilateral leg complaints. A Doppler ultrasound was requested by her family physician given the likelihood for venous thrombosis. She was otherwise healthy and had started oral contraception a few weeks ago. The ultrasound con-

**Table 1** Case scenarios in this chapter

| CASE | Issue | Key points |
|---|---|---|
| Case 1 | Concomitant deep venous thrombosis (DVT) and pulmonary embolism (PE) | PE confirmation with CTA not always necessary |
| Case 2 | PE false positive and PE rule-out criteria (PERC) score missing | PERC help rule out PE in patients <50 years old |
| Case 3 | Acute dyspnea in the patient already anticoagulated | Heart failure underdiagnosis |
| Case 4 | IVC filter: Interventional radiology (IR) or surgery? | Better outcomes with IR expertise input |
| Case 5 | Preoperative cardiac CT/MRI | Coronary artery calcification (CAC) score never needed |
| Case 6 | Chest pain in ED | Coronary CTA very valuable |

firmed popliteal vein thrombosis. The next appointment for her family physician was within 3 days, to discuss the imaging results. Meanwhile, 2 days after having undergone ultrasound she developed localized pleuritic chest pain and decided to go to the hospital ED. A chest CTA was requested.

## 2.1 Role of Imaging: A Value-Based Approach

In case of suspected DVT the first step should be to assess the clinical probability with the well-known two-level DVT Wells score (Wells et al. 2003). If the score gives *likely*, then the patient should proceed to ultrasound to confirm or exclude that diagnosis. If the score gives *unlikely*, then D-dimer testing is the next step, somewhat similar to PE diagnosis (Di Nisio et al. 2016). In this way, DVT can be safely ruled out and imaging safely omitted in a patient who has an *unlikely* Wells score for DVT and a negative D-dimer test. If D-dimer is positive, then an ultrasound should be requested (Wells et al. 2003; Di Nisio et al. 2016). Not to be confused, the Wells score for PE (Wells et al. 2000) and the simplified version of this Wells score for PE (Gibson et al. 2008) are different item blocks of clinical criteria comparatively to that for DVT.

Our straightforward case scenario for a female patient with confirmed proximal DVT and concomitant development of PE given a very likely clot migration with peripheral lung infarct is emblematic of how pure reliance on guidelines or clinical decision support (CDS) tools could be tricky. No doubt that in our case scenario, applying PE diagnostic algorithm or a CDS software with ACR Appropriateness Criteria and, once requested, a chest CTA would be considered appropriate, but …

### 2.1.1 Is This Chest CTA Really Necessary?

It has been stated that for suspected PE, a diagnosis of proximal DVT in a symptomatic patient (as in our case scenario) is considered sufficient to rule in and treat PE (Goldhaber and Bounameaux 2012). More recently, different authors also state that, especially when it is desirable to avoid CTA (e.g., pregnancy, youngs, renal failure), ultrasound-proven proximal DVT alone is considered sufficient to rule in PE and initiate the respective treatment (Hirmerova et al. 2018; Konstantinides et al. 2014). In this regard, one should also remember that ATS-STR guideline clearly considers chest CTA as a second line in the diagnostic workup for PE in pregnancy. Although lung scintigraphy and chest CTA have both roughly equivalent dose as that absorbed by the fetus from naturally occurring background radiation during a 9-month period, the maternal dose in CTA is much higher than that from the scintigraphy (namely to the lung and breast) (Leung et al. 2011). Moreover, if no difference in medical treatment exists between a simple proximal DVT with or without a concomitant simple PE (that is, a low- or very-low-risk PESI score, hemodynamically stable patient with neither laboratorial nor echo evidence of right ventricular strain), it is appropriate to refrain from ordering a pulmonary CTA (Kearon et al. 2016; Wilbur and Shian 2017). ESC guidelines clearly support avoidance of CTA in pregnancy, once DVT is confirmed, stating that it already warrants anticoagulation treatment (Konstantinides et al. 2014). The American College of Physicians (ACP), in their best practice recommendations on PE released in 2015, also states that in the hemodynamically stable patient (irrespective of age or pregnancy), an ultrasound should be sufficient. If a DVT is confirmed, the need for anticoagulation will also be established, and a similar treatment will be pursued without exposing the patient to the risks of iodinated contrast or ionizing radiation (Raja et al. 2015).

Furthermore, safe outpatient treatment for simple low-risk PE is gaining momentum, as it also has proved efficacy in simple DVT (Kearon et al. 2016; Wilbur and Shian 2017).

The other way round—screening for DVT with ultrasound in the setting of acute PE diagnosed by imaging—seems to be justified because of:

– A high incidence of asymptomatic DVT and a high risk of subsequent development of post-thrombotic syndrome—in this way, prophylaxis or a timely preventive strategic plan could be set in advance (Hirmerova et al. 2018).

– The importance of deciding whether or not to anticoagulate the low-risk patient with an isolated subsegmental PE (Fig. 1)—if a DVT is depicted, logically yes; if DVT is excluded, no (Kearon et al. 2016).

**Key Points**
- **Value-driven clinical decision:** Do not rely solely on guidelines or CDS tools. Always reflect the individual clinical situation. Make the diagnosis and treat with minimum resources as possible, maintaining the best outcome: increase value.
- **Reduce redundancy, reduce costs:** DVT can be safely ruled out and imaging safely omitted in a patient who has an *unlikely* Wells score for DVT and a negative D-dimer test.
- **Isolated subsegmental PE:** Clinical surveillance is preferred over anticoagulation in low-risk patients once no DVT is depicted on US.

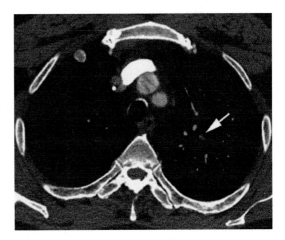

**Fig. 1** A subsegmental PE is depicted in this companion case. If isolated, usually it is an incidental finding of questionable significance [reprinted by permission from Springer Nature: Kallen, J.A., Coughlin, B.F., O'Loughlin, M.T. et al. *Reduced Z-axis coverage multidetector CT angiography for suspected acute pulmonary embolism could decrease dose and maintain diagnostic accuracy.* Emerg Radiol (2010) 17: 31–5. Doi: 10.1007/s10140-009-0818-6]

## 3    Case 2: Pulmonary Embolism

A 32-year-old female with a recent onset of periscapular pain radiating to the back was observed in the ED. She also complained of breathlessness while waiting in the ED. She was otherwise healthy as stated in the request form for a chest CTA to check the possibility of PE as the D-dimer test came out positive. The CTA was reported as positive for PE, by an outsourced teleradiology company at night. The patient was admitted and 2 days later the internal medicine physician asks for an attending radiologist's second opinion about the CTA report, as he feels there is, at least currently, some clinical incongruence for PE.

### 3.1    Role of Imaging: A Value-Based Approach

The value of a radiology consultation service or the on-site presence of an attending radiologist cannot be overemphasized. In this case, after reviewing the images from the chest CTA requested in the ED, the attending radiologist concluded that it was a false-positive report with a respiratory motion artifact mimicking PE. It is well known that the false-positive rate for PE is higher than the false-negative rate. Other common causes for false positives include cardiac pulsation, poor pulmonary arterial opacification from Valsalva maneuver or contrast material mixing, attenuation artifact due to beam hardening, or adjacent airspace disease (Hutchinson et al. 2015).

#### 3.1.1    The Caveat of a Positive D-Dimer Test

In the multidisciplinary discussion, the radiologist and the internal medicine physician retrospectively reviewed all the previous electronic medical records (EMR) from that patient, and concluded that actually she was not so "otherwise healthy": she had past history of anxiety and was being regularly followed in the psychosomatic consult. Nevertheless, the CTA request could have been seen as appropriate according to the most used guidelines as well as to the ACR

Appropriateness Criteria used in the most popular CDS tools nowadays (Konstantinides et al. 2014; American College of Radiology Appropriateness Criteria® 2018) because this patient had low probability score but a positive D-dimer test (cf. Table 2).

The problem is that PERC score is not yet universally adopted or integrated into most well-known algorithms for PE diagnostic workup. It has been used with some variability across different institutions since its inception, more than a decade ago (Kline et al. 2004). In our case scenario the radiologist raised that possibility and all the items necessary to calculate this score were shown retrospectively to be available in the EMR from this acute episode of care: the score was zero.

The ACP best practice advice on PE diagnostic workup already includes a clear indication for not testing D-dimer nor requesting imaging studies in patients with a low pretest probability of PE and a PERC score of zero (Raja et al. 2015). Very recently, the groundbreaking French PROPER trial (noninferiority, crossover, and cluster-randomized) shed more light on the efficacy of the PERC score and seemed to definitively refute some concerns on feasibility across different countries or continents (Freund et al. 2018). As such, a more widespread inclusion of the PERC score into updated guidelines from different societies and associations can be expected.

In conclusion, this case scenario once again emphasizes that value-based radiology requires much more than a simple adherence to CDS tools. An appropriate request does not mean that the request is needed in the individual clinical setting, if one wants to avoid redundancy, potential harm, and costs. The series of unfortunate events experienced by the patient (missed PERC score followed by CTA false positive for PE) also point toward the value of an attending radiologist present at the institution and a good IT

**Table 2** Common causes for the frequently found positive D-dimer test

| Infection | Trauma/injury | Liver disease |
|---|---|---|
| Inflammation | Recent surgery | Renal/heart failure |
| Malignancy | Pregnancy | Ageing |

infrastructure providing fast access to the clinic notes in the EMR (Mongan and Avrin 2018).

---

**Key Points**

- **Value of second opinion by subspecialty radiology:** A review by an experienced thoracic radiologist is strongly encouraged in cases of low burden or equivocal PE imaging (Pena et al. 2012).
- **PERC score:** Should be actively pursued in patients <50 years old, because an age >49 years instantly adds 1 point to the score not precluding the need for D-dimer testing (Raja et al. 2015).
- **Value of efficient PACS-EMR integration:** A fast way to consult additional clinical information is of utmost importance for the radiologist, to bring added value in a MDT discussion and increase the awareness for missing data (e.g., the PERC score in our case scenario).

---

## 4    Case 3: Dyspnea of Cardiac Origin

A 64-year-old male presents with shortness of breath in the ED. He had a past history of aortic valve replacement and his current INR was 2.8. Atrial fibrillation was revealed by ECG. Lab tests showed that D-dimer was positive. During overnight, the ED doctor wanted to call the radiologist about a chest CTA request. This was not possible because the radiology service was outsourced for teleradiology. Nevertheless, he felt comfortable when the CDS software indicated "Appropriate" while clicking on the contrast-enhanced chest CTA option for suspected PE due to the positive D-dimer test.

## 4.1    Role of Imaging: A Value-Based Approach

As the D-dimer test is very sensitive but with low specificity, a positive value in this case scenario should be interpreted somewhat the same way in the last case (missed PERC score). Levels of as

high as 22% of positive D-dimer tests could be seen in patients on anticoagulant therapy, with no recurrent PE at all (Vorobyeva et al. 2013). In 2008, Meyer et al. analyzed the results of six randomized controlled trials including 5461 patients and reported a PE rate of 3.3% (Meyer et al. 2008), although not describing how many were adequately anticoagulated. More recently, in the era of multi-detector CT (MDCT), Liu et al. found a rate of 1.2% among a total of 2996 patients. Interestingly, half of these patients with breakthrough PE had at least one subtherapeutic INR (<2.0) in the preceding 2 weeks (Liu et al. 2018). Furthermore, both studies assessed neither the possibility of false-positive CT scans nor the prevalence of isolated subsegmental PE.

It is worth remembering the frequent overdiagnosis PE by general radiologists compared to dedicated thoracic radiologists (Hutchinson et al. 2015). False-positive rates as high as 42% have been described by Stein et al. (2006). Furthermore, the rate of isolated subsegmental PE has steeply increased in the era of MDCT, with a clear propensity to overdiagnosis, reaching values as high as 15% (Wiener et al. 2013; Carrier et al. 2010).

## 4.2    Dyspnea of Cardiac Origin

In case of dyspnea of suspected cardiac origin, the imaging investigation should start with chest X-ray (CXR) as in suspected pulmonary origin. CXR is top rated (9 points) by ACR (American College of Radiology Appropriateness Criteria® 2018) in all the five cardiac scenarios:

- Heart failure (HF) with possible ischemia.
- Heart failure with ischemia excluded.
- Arrhythmia/valvular heart disease/pericardial disease, all with ischemia excluded.

Transthoracic echocardiography is also rated at the same level for these five scenarios (American College of Radiology Appropriateness Criteria® 2018).

### 4.2.1    Heart Failure

It is well stated in literature that HF is widely underdiagnosed, especially in the first acute episodes as well as in older people (van Riet et al. 2014; Marx 2017). In diabetes type 2, HF is the second most common initial manifestation of cardiovascular disease, just behind peripheral arterial disease. Angina, myocardial infarction, or stroke are less frequent as recently shown by Shah et al. (2015).

The pivotal Doppler findings in echo to diagnose diastolic dysfunction or HF with preserved ejection fraction (HFpEF) are often missing. The reasons can be manifold: lack of awareness, expertise, availability, or reimbursement. However, it is important to remember that HFpEF constitutes approximately 50% of the cases of HF, and frequent triggers for acute exacerbations are uncontrolled hypertension and atrial fibrillation, as in our case scenario (Oktay and Shah 2015; Ponikowski et al. 2016).

If all the clinical data, the sometimes subtle findings of HF at CXR, and the Doppler evidence of diastolic dysfunction (Fig. 2) are not adequately put all together, this important diagnosis might be frequently missed. At the same time referring physicians might request CT to rule out PE or identify different reasons that might point towards the cause of dyspnea.

Having said that, one must also reflect on the last-decade fivefold rise in CT requests for PE (Venkatesh et al. 2018), and the resulting low levels of diagnostic yield for PE, that varies between 6% (Venkatesh et al. 2018) and 15% (Chong et al. 2018; Chung et al. 2018). In Table 3 other common causes for dyspnea are displayed. These might be frequently overlooked and could be more or less easily diagnosed with clinical and

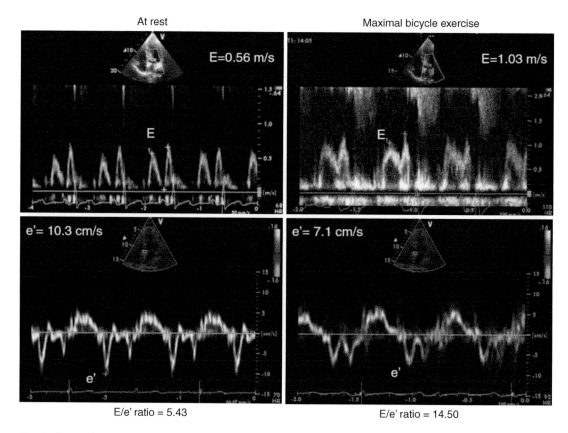

**Fig. 2** Companion case of a patient with effort dyspnea and evidence of diastolic dysfunction only on stress/exercise: Key functional alterations (most used cutoff values) are an E/e′ ≥13 and a mean e′ septal and lateral wall <9 cm/s (Ponikowski et al. 2016) [reprinted by permission from Springer Nature: Galderisi M., Picano E. (2015) Diastolic Stress Echocardiography. In: Stress Echocardiography. Springer, Cham. Doi: 10.1007/978-3-319-20,958-6_25]

**Table 3** Common causes for dyspnea/breathlessness, besides PE, frequently overlooked in ED

| Heart failure | Pneumonia | TRALI |
|---|---|---|
| Alveolar edema | Lymphangitic carcinomatosis | Pleural effusion |
| ARDS | | Pneumothorax |

Abbreviations: *ARDS* acute respiratory distress syndrome, *TRALI* transfusion-related acute lung injury

laboratorial data, aided with CXR and US/echo, only complemented by CT if the earlier workup was inconclusive.

---

**Key Points: The problematic of PE and CTA**
- **Inefficiency in CTA use:** A fivefold increase in the use was seen in the last decade, while the diagnostic yield has remained low, with negative rates of 85–94%.
- **High rates of PE false positives:** In 6–15% of cases CTA is positive for PE; however up to 42% might be false positives—due to artifacts, non-subspecialty CTA reading, etc.—as well as 15% might be isolated subsegmental PE of questionable clinical significance.
- **Non-incorporation of PERC rules:** Most guidelines or algorithms in CDS tools lack yet the added value of PERC score in ruling out PE in patients <50 years old.
- **Breakthrough PE:** If a negative predictive value of 99% is already used to safely rule out PE in a patient with negative D-dimer, there is no reason to investigate further the <1% rate of breakthrough PE in an adequately anticoagulated patient.

---

# 5    Case 4: IVC Filter

A 55-year-old male presented with abdominal pain for some weeks. He had a past history of IVC filter placement some months ago in a vascular surgery facility. An abdominal CT was requested to clarify the patient complaints, and the requesting physician asks for a radiologist's second opinion as potential complications of the IVC filter were not reported.

## 5.1    Role of Imaging: A Value-Based Approach

A long indwell time for IVC filter is a risk factor for complications related with this device. Described complications involve more frequently: penetration of adjacent organ (Fig. 3), fracture, migration, or thrombus-related complications such as caval thrombosis or stenosis (Angel et al. 2011; Shin et al. 2018; Juluru et al. 2018).

Many of these complications are frequently overlooked or not reported. Also, even if reported, the lack of a proper mechanism of notification to the requesting physician could result in mismanagement (Shin et al. 2018). In this regard, Shin et al. have recently shown in a retrospective analysis, the added value of structured reporting for IVC filters in abdominal CT reports. The rate of reported complications increased from 12% (before the implementation) to 57% (after) (Shin et al. 2018).

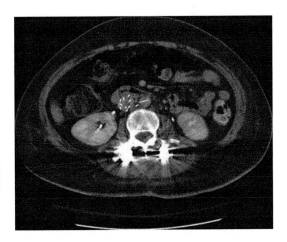

**Fig. 3** Companion case showing migration of the limbs of an inferior vena cava filter, where a strut is seen crossing the aorta [reprinted by permission from Springer Nature: Clark S., Rodriguez H.E. (2014) Retrievable Inferior Vena Cava (IVC) Filters. In: Dieter R., Dieter, Jr. R., Dieter, III R. (eds) Endovascular Interventions. Springer, New York, NY. Doi: 10.1007/978-1-4,614-7,312-1_88]

As a suggestion, one could add to the local or personal armamentarium of templates, something like the examples shown below:

– The IVC filter is depicted in [infrarenal/suprarenal] location. No evidence of strut fracture, organ penetration, or organ involvement.
– The IVC filter is depicted in [infrarenal/suprarenal] location. The following findings are present: [fracture/penetration/clot or other/free text].

The problem with patient follow-up, retrieval scheduling, and peer communication between the different physicians for patients with IVC filters was also addressed elegantly in the study by Juluru et al. (2018). In their work, they have developed a software application, integrated in the hospital network that tracks patients with IVC filters, making the process of proper longitudinal coordinated care much easier. Increased rates of filter retrieval, better communication between interventional radiology (IR) team and referrers, and better workflow in visit scheduling were shown (Juluru et al. 2018).

Furthermore, better outcomes for the patient and reduced costs are described for IVC filter procedures in the setting of IR compared to surgery or even interventional cardiology (Makary et al. 2018). The recent study by Makary et al. showed lesser postprocedural complications for IVC filter placement, higher success rates in retrieval, and lower fluoroscopy times (Makary et al. 2018).

> **Key Points**
> • **The added value of IR in IVC filter management:** Expertise input in macros development for CT report and in management software for follow-up and tracking of patients with IVC filters. Better outcomes and reduced costs compared to surgery or interventional cardiology.

## 6 Case 5: Coronary Artery Calcium Scoring and Stress Cardiac MR

A CT for CAC scoring and a stress CMR were requested by the anesthesiologist for preoperative assessment (cholecystectomy) of a 59-year-old man who had a past history of cardiac disease. The interview and physical examination confirmed currently no symptoms and stable condition, but the patient didn't recall the precise type of "cardiac disease" he had been diagnosed 3 years ago by the cardiologist.

### 6.1 Role of Imaging: A Value-Based Approach

The value of a good IT infrastructure providing fast access to past patient information in the EMR cannot be overemphasized. The rapid retrieval of information, like previous coronary stents or bypass grafts, would immediately point towards a precise cardiac disease—coronary artery disease (CAD)—that would preclude the request of a CAC score. Also, even if a cardiomyopathy or a valvular disease were found, CAC score is considered inappropriate in a preoperative evaluation, irrespective of the patient risk (Choosing Wisely® 2018).

CAC score is also not recommended for screening purposes, even in a non-preoperative evaluation, for the asymptomatic low-risk patient, except if a familiar history of premature CAD is known (Choosing Wisely® 2018). Recently, USPSTF has even concluded for insufficient evidence for the added value of CAC score in addition to the traditional risk assessment for cardiovascular diseases (CVD) in asymptomatic patients to prevent CVD events (US Preventive Services Task Force et al. 2018).

Regarding the stress testing, both the American Society for Anesthesiologists (ASA) and Society for Cardiovascular Magnetic Resonance (SCMR) recommendations in *Choosing Wisely* are convergent: in low- or moderate-risk noncardiac surgery (cf. Table 4), cardiac stress testing is not recommended for the

**Table 4** Examples of low-, moderate-, and high-risk noncardiac surgeries

| Low risk | Moderate risk | High risk |
|---|---|---|
| Small parts | Common abdominal (GI/GU/GYN) | Lung/liver transplant |
| Breast/thyroid | | Aortic/major vascular surgery |
| Eye/dental | Neurological/Orthop. | |

stable asymptomatic patient even with a known cardiac disease (Choosing Wisely® 2018).

## 6.2 Rationale

The purpose of a preoperative evaluation in cardiac patients is to detect conditions that would change pre- or peri-surgical management (decreasing the risk to the patient) or even change the decision of the patient to undergo surgery. In this regard, one must bear in mind that the indications to submit a patient to a preoperative revascularization are similar to those as in a non-surgical setting (Velasco et al. 2017), that is, in appropriate clinical scenarios with clear symptoms or signs of ischemia/infarction usually coupled with supportive ECG and laboratorial evidence.

A categorical class III recommendation (no benefit/possible harm) is provided by the latest ESC/ESA guideline for elective revascularization before low- and intermediate-risk surgeries in patients with known CAD, prior to noncardiac surgery (Velasco et al. 2017).

So, in our case scenario, even if CAD and/or stress perfusion alterations were shown, that wouldn't change the pre-surgical management (e.g., a putative elective revascularization) and the patient could safely proceed to his intermediate-risk noncardiac surgery (cholecystectomy).

In a study about the overuse of preoperative cardiac stress testing, Sheffield et al. found a nearly fourfold increase, between 1996 and 2007, in patients with no cardiac indications having preoperative stress testing. Interestingly, they showed that patients who were more likely to undergo preoperative stress testing lived in areas with more cardiologists per 100,000 (Sheffield et al. 2013), emphasizing once again the

drawbacks of the self-referrals and the fee-for-service model.

> **Key Points**
> - **CAC score:** Not recommended for patients neither with known CAD nor for preoperative assessment in any surgery, whatever the risk of patient is.
> - **Stress (CMR) testing:** In low- or moderate-risk noncardiac surgery, cardiac stress testing in not recommended for the stable asymptomatic patient even with a known past history of cardiac disease.

## 7 Case 6: Coronary CTA in the ED

A 62-year-old male was brought to the ED complaining of chest pain. After initial clinical evaluation complemented with ECG and troponin, the overall findings neither completely ruled in nor ruled out an acute coronary syndrome (ACS). The ED physician decided to consult the institutional CDS tool for "Chest Pain Suggestive of Acute Coronary Syndrome" based on the ACR Appropriateness Criteria and ordered a radionuclide myocardial perfusion imaging (MPI) test because it was displayed as the top-rated exam.

### 7.1 Role of Imaging: A Value-Based Approach

This case scenario illustrates the possible drawbacks of pure reliance on CDS tools, as it could sometimes be misleading. In this particular example, the ACR Appropriateness Criteria currently displayed on website (American College of Radiology Appropriateness Criteria® 2018) are not up to date (last revision made in 2014). A very recent paper by Levin et al. (2018) clearly flags this caveat in ACR Appropriateness Criteria regarding chest pain suggestive of ACS, stating that it should be revised to rate coronary CTA higher than nuclear MPI or stress echo, given the huge amount of evidence that was published in the last years.

Interestingly in 2015, a joint committee/task force, representing many medical societies (ACR being the head), published a guideline for appropriate utilization of cardiovascular imaging for patients presenting with chest pain in ED (Rybicki et al. 2016). Among 20 clinical scenarios of chest pain—encompassing diagnosis like clear-cut ACS, possible ACS, chest pain of noncardiac cause, PE, and acute aortic syndromes—in 6 of them coronary CTA was considered clearly appropriate, namely:

1. Troponin initially equivocal/single-troponin elevation, and no additional evidence of ACS.
2. Symptoms of ischemia have resolved hours before ECG/lab/echo testing.
3. Patients with TIMI (thrombolysis in myocardial infarction) risk score of 0, early high sensitivity troponins negative.
4. Initial ECG normal or nonischemic, normal initial troponin.
5. Observational pathway with serial ECG and troponins negative, but possible unstable angina.
6. Observational pathway with serial ECG or troponins borderline for ACS.

The first four clinical scenarios integrate the early assessment pathway, where other imaging exams such as rest SPECT/CMR/echo vary in their rating of appropriateness between "rarely appropriate" and "may be appropriate," while coronary CTA is considered top-rated as stated above: the only clearly appropriate (Rybicki et al. 2016).

The observational pathway (last two clinical scenarios) constitutes, alongside the fourth clinical scenario, a big proportion of patients seen in the ED with chest pain suggestive of ACS. In this observational pathway scenarios stress SPECT/CMR/echo are regarded as clearly appropriate at the same level as coronary CTA (Rybicki et al. 2016).

## 7.2 Rationale

Three recent trials have shown that coronary CTA is effective and advantageous for patients presenting in the ED with acute chest pain. CT-STAT trial was the first to show that in low-risk patients with chest pain, the use of coronary CTA resulted in a faster diagnosis comparatively to radionuclide MPI and was associated with lower total ED costs (a median total ED cost of $2137 vs. $3,458 in the MPI cohort, that is, 38% lower) (Goldstein et al. 2011). With similar safety (regarding incidence of subsequent major adverse cardiac events) and a statistically significant lower radiation burden comparatively to MPI, the coronary CTA strategy was able to reach a diagnosis within a median time of 2.9 vs. 6.2 h in the MPI cohort (54% reduction) (Goldstein et al. 2011).

The second trial (five-center, randomized) published in 2012 by Litt et al. (2012) broadened the scope, including not just low- but also intermediate-risk patients because overall they accounted for nearly 50–70% of presentations with a possible ACS. They found that patients in the coronary CTA group had also a shorter median length of stay (18 vs. 25 h in the traditional care arm), and a higher rate of discharge directly from the ED (50 vs. 23%). In either cohort, there were no deaths within 30 days after presentation and the same incidence of 1% in myocardial infarction was shown (Litt et al. 2012).

ROMICAT II, the third trial, nine-center and randomized, published in 2012 (Hoffmann et al. 2012), again compared coronary CTA versus standard of care and found that triage in the ED had an improved efficiency in the CTA cohort. Again a shorter median length of stay (9 vs. 27 h) and more frequent direct discharge from the ED were shown (47 vs. 12%). Regarding the safety, again no significant differences in major adverse cardiovascular events were seen at the end of 4 weeks in both groups. Interestingly, in this study no differences in costs were shown, because in the standard care group only a minority of patients underwent MPI (majority got only stress echo or stress test without imaging) (Hoffmann et al. 2012).

Bottom line, the British NICE guideline on chest pain of recent onset has been recently updated in November 2016 (National Institute for Health and Care Excellence 2018), including a recommendation of a first-line coronary CTA for:

- All patients, without established CAD who present with recent onset of chest pain with typical or atypical anginal features.
- Patients with non-anginal chest pain of recent onset, but an abnormal resting ECG (ST-T changes or Q waves).

> **Key Points**
> - **Coronary CTA:** Should be considered as the test of choice in most patients without known CAD, presenting with chest pain suggestive but not diagnostic of ACS. Its safety, accuracy, and cost-effectiveness have been shown in various randomized clinical trials.
> - **CDS tools:** Should be regularly updated/audited internally by institutionally approved multidisciplinary board, as outdated versions and its use without critical judgment could be misleading.

## 8 Summary

Radiologists can add value to different episodes of care, either through outcome improvement (IVC filter management by IR, better tracking of patients with radiology-developed software, and structured reporting for CT; early safe discharge from ED of patients with chest pain by coronary

CTA testing; etc.) or through avoidance of redundant or inappropriate imaging—e.g., pulmonary CTA in patients with a PERC score of zero, already adequately anticoagulated and where the clinical, analytic, and basic imaging picture is already straightforward for another diagnosis than PE.

As cardiovascular imaging is an ever-evolving field, with constant update in different societal guidelines and ever-new groundbreaking trials, one must be very cautious when using CDS tools without a critical thinking as they might be misleading (not up to date, somewhat confusing or with apparent conflicting algorithms at first glance for the inexperienced requesting clinician). Different local practices have to be taken into consideration, and teamwork in multidisciplinary setting is of pivotal importance, because only a team working on the same lane with a value-driven mindset will achieve the highest value in the episode of care, either through increase in outcomes (the equation numerator) or through cost reduction (the equation denominator). Turf battles or resistance to adhere to guideline or to accept the advice from the radiologist will perpetuate the issue of low-value care, either for a worse rate of complications in IVC filter retrieval in a non-IR setting or for the maintenance of unacceptably high rates of negative pulmonary CTA, etc.

## References

American College of Radiology Appropriateness Criteria® (2018). https://www.acr.org/Clinical-Resources/ACR-Appropriateness-Criteria. Accessed 30 Aug 2018

Angel LF, Tapson V, Galgon RE et al (2011) Systematic review of the use of retrievable inferior vena cava filters. J Vasc Interv Radiol 22(11):1522–1530.e3

Carrier M, Righini M, Wells PS et al (2010) Subsegmental pulmonary embolism diagnosed by computed tomography: incidence and clinical implications. A systematic review and meta-analysis of the management outcome studies. J Thromb Haemost 8:1716–1722

Chong J, Lee TC, Attarian A et al (2018) Association of lower diagnostic yield with high users of CT pulmonary angiogram. JAMA Intern Med 178(3):412–413

Choosing Wisely® (2018). The American Board of Internal Medicine Foundation. http://www.

choosingwisely.org/wp-content/uploads/2015/01/ Choosing-Wisely-Recommendations.pdf. Accessed 30 Aug 2018

Chung JH, Landeras L, Haas K et al (2018) The value of a disease-specific template and an IT-based quality tracking system in pulmonary embolism CT angiography. J Am Coll Radiol 15(7):988–992

Di Nisio M, van Es N, Büller HR (2016) Deep vein thrombosis and pulmonary embolism. Lancet 388(10063):3060–3073

Freund Y, Cachanado M, Aubry A et al (2018) Effect of the pulmonary embolism rule-out criteria on subsequent thromboembolic events among low-risk emergency department patients: the PROPER randomized clinical trial. JAMA 319(6):559–566

Gibson NS, Sohne M, Kruip MJ et al (2008) Further validation and simplification of the Wells clinical decision rule in pulmonary embolism. Thromb Haemost 99:229–234

Goldhaber SZ, Bounameaux H (2012) Pulmonary embolism and deep vein thrombosis. Lancet 379(9828):1835–1846

Goldstein JA, Chinnaiyan KM, Abidov A et al (2011) The CT-STAT (coronary computed tomographic angiography for systematic triage of acute chest pain patients to treatment) trial. J Am Coll Cardiol 58:1414–1422

Hirmerova J, Seidlerova J, Chudacek Z (2018) The prevalence of concomitant deep vein thrombosis, symptomatic or asymptomatic, proximal or distal, in patients with symptomatic pulmonary embolism. Clin Appl Thromb Hemost 24(8):1352–1357

Hoffmann U, Truong QA, Schoenfeld DA et al (2012) Coronary CT angiography versus standard evaluation in acute chest pain. N Engl J Med 367:299–308

Hutchinson BD, Navin P, Marom EM et al (2015) Overdiagnosis of pulmonary embolism by pulmonary CT angiography. AJR Am J Roentgenol 205(2):271–277

Juluru K, Elnajjar P, Shih HH et al (2018) An informatics approach to facilitate clinical management of patients with retrievable inferior vena cava filters. AJR Am J Roentgenol 5:W1–W7

Kearon C, Akl EA, Ornelas J et al (2016) Antithrombotic therapy for VTE disease: CHEST guideline and expert panel report. Chest 149:315–352

Kline JA, Mitchell AM, Kabrhel C et al (2004) Clinical criteria to prevent unnecessary diagnostic testing in emergency department patients with suspected pulmonary embolism. J Thromb Haemost 2(8):1247–1255

Konstantinides SV, Torbicki A, Agnelli G et al (2014) ESC guidelines on the diagnosis and management of acute pulmonary embolism. Eur Heart J 35(43): 3033–3069, 3069a–3069k

Leung AN, Bull TM, Jaeschke R et al (2011) An official American Thoracic Society/Society of Thoracic Radiology clinical practice guideline: evaluation of suspected pulmonary embolism in pregnancy. Am J Respir Crit Care Med 184(10):1200–1208

Levin DC, Parker L, Halpern EJ et al (2018) Coronary CT angiography: use in patients with chest pain presenting to emergency departments. AJR Am J Roentgenol 210(4):816–820

Litt HI, Gatsonis C, Snyder B et al (2012) CT angiography for safe discharge of patients with possible acute coronary syndromes. N Engl J Med 366:1393–1403

Liu MY, Ballard DW, Huang J et al (2018) Acute pulmonary embolism in emergency department patients despite therapeutic anticoagulation. West J Emerg Med 19(3):510–516

Makary MS, Kapke J, Yildiz V et al (2018) Outcomes and direct costs of inferior vena cava filter placement and retrieval within the IR and surgical settings. J Vasc Interv Radiol 29(2):170–175

Marx N (2017) Heart failure and diabetes - underestimated, underdiagnosed and poorly understood: a call for action. Diab Vasc Dis Res 14(2):67–68

Meyer G, Planquette B, Sanchez O (2008) Long-term outcome of pulmonary embolism. Curr Opin Hematol 15(5):499–503

Mongan J, Avrin D (2018) Impact of PACS-EMR integration on radiologist usage of the EMR. J Digit Imaging 31(5):611–614. https://doi.org/10.1007/s10278-018-0077-8

National Institute for Health and Care Excellence (2018). Chest pain of recent onset: assessment and diagnosis. https://www.nice.org.uk/guidance/cg95. Accessed 30 Aug 2018

Oktay AA, Shah SJ (2015) Diagnosis and management of heart failure with preserved ejection fraction: 10 key lessons. Curr Cardiol Rev 11(1):42–52

Pena E, Kimpton M, Dennie C et al (2012) Difference in interpretation of computed tomography pulmonary angiography diagnosis of subsegmental thrombosis in patients with suspected pulmonary embolism. J Thromb Haemost 10(3):496–498

Ponikowski P, Voors AA, Anker SD et al (2016) 2016 ESC guidelines for the diagnosis and treatment of acute and chronic heart failure. Eur J Heart Fail 18(8): 891–975

Raja AS, Greenberg JO, Qaseem A et al (2015) Evaluation of patients with suspected acute pulmonary embolism: best practice advice from the clinical guidelines Committee of the American College of physicians. Ann Intern Med 163(9):701–711

Rybicki FJ, Udelson JE, Peacock WF et al (2016) Appropriate utilization of cardiovascular imaging in emergency department patients with chest pain. J Am Coll Radiol 13(2):e1–e29

Shah AD, Langenberg C, Rapsomaniki E et al (2015) Type 2 diabetes and incidence of cardiovascular diseases: a cohort study in 1·9 million people. Lancet Diabetes Endocrinol 3(2):105–113

Sheffield KM, McAdams PS, Benarroch-Gampel J et al (2013) Overuse of preoperative cardiac stress testing in Medicare patients undergoing elective noncardiac surgery. Ann Surg 257(1):73–80

Shin BJ, Habibollahi P, Zafar H et al (2018) Reporting of inferior vena cava filter complications on CT: impact of standardized macros. AJR Am J Roentgenol 211(2):439–444

Stein PD, Fowler SE, Goodman LR et al (2006) Multidetector computed tomography for acute pulmonary embolism. N Engl J Med 354:2317–2327

US Preventive Services Task Force, Curry SJ, Krist AH, Owens DK et al (2018) Risk assessment for cardiovascular disease with nontraditional risk factors: US preventive services task force recommendation statement. JAMA 320(3):272–280

van Riet EES, Hoes AW, Limburg A et al (2014) Prevalence of unrecognized heart failure in older persons with shortness of breath on exertion. Eur J Heart Fail 16(7):772–777

Velasco A, Reyes E, Hage FG (2017) Guidelines in review: comparison of the 2014 ACC/AHA guidelines on perioperative cardiovascular evaluation and management of patients undergoing noncardiac surgery and the 2014 ESC/ESA guidelines on noncardiac surgery: cardiovascular assessment and management. J Nucl Cardiol 24(1):165–170

Venkatesh AK, Agha L, Abaluck J et al (2018) Trends and variation in the utilization and diagnostic yield of chest imaging for medicare patients with suspected pulmonary embolism in the emergency department. AJR Am J Roentgenol 210(3):572–577

Vorobyeva NM, Dobrovolsky AB, Titaeva EV, Kirienko AI, Panchenko EP (2013) D-dimer testing during anticoagulant therapy should be used to indicate patients who need extended anticoagulant therapy. Eur Heart J 34(suppl_1):1080. https://doi.org/10.1093/eurheartj/eht308.1080

Wells PS, Anderson DR, Rodger M et al (2000) Derivation of a simple clinical model to categorize patients probability of pulmonary embolism: increasing the models utility with the SimpliRED D-dimer. Thromb Haemost 83:416–420

Wells PS, Anderson DR, Rodger M et al (2003) Evaluation of D-dimer in the diagnosis of suspected deep-vein thrombosis. N Engl J Med 349:1227–1235

Wiener RS, Schwartz LM, Woloshin S (2013) When a test is too good: how CT pulmonary angiograms find pulmonary emboli that do not need to be found. BMJ 347:f3368

Wilbur J, Shian B (2017) Deep venous thrombosis and pulmonary embolism: current therapy. Am Fam Physician 95(5):295–302

Printed in the United States
By Bookmasters